Burn Calories While You Sleep

Change Your Metabolism to be Thin, Fit, Healthy, and Live Longer

by

Tim A. Fischell, M.D.

Foreword by Dean Ornish, M.D.

Brighton Publishing LLC
501 W. Ray Road
Suite 4
Chandler, AZ 85225
www.BrightonPublishing.com

Burn Calories While You Sleep

Change Your Metabolism to be Thin, Fit, Healthy, and Live Longer

by

Tim A. Fischell, M.D.

Foreword by Dean Ornish, M.D.

Brighton Publishing LLC
501 W. Ray Road
Suite 4
Chandler, AZ 85225
www.BrightonPublishing.com

First Edition

Printed in the United States of America

ISBN 13: 978-1-621830-51-1
ISBN 10: 1-62183051-9
Cover Design: Tom Rodriguez

❧ *Dedication* ❧

Dedicated to my family, and in memory of my wonderful mother Marian and my dearest friend Michael Land.

❧ *Foreword* ❧

by

DEAN ORNISH, M.D.

Founder & President, Preventive Medicine Research Institute Clinical Professor of Medicine, University of California, San Francisco. Author of: The Spectrum and Dr. Dean Ornish's Program for Reversing Heart Disease

In this book, Dr. Tim Fischell describes a comprehensive lifestyle program—a time-efficient and sustainable way of exercising, eating and living that helps you lose weight, keep it off, and enhances your health rather than harming it.

Tim and I completed our internship and residency together in internal medicine many years ago at the Massachusetts General Hospital and Harvard Medical School. When you spend three years together with someone in such extreme circumstances, you see clearly who they are and what they're really like.

I was always impressed with Tim's intelligence, creativity, and fearlessness, as well as his kindness. He went on to become one of the country's leading interventional cardiologists— clinically outstanding and highly regarded as a clinician, teacher and researcher. He has published more than one-hundred papers in peer-reviewed journals. As a scientist, he understands the differences between fads and interventions based on the scientific method.

He is also an innovative inventor who has been issued nearly one hundred patents in the field of medical device technologies. He has applied many of these same inventive skills in developing a lifestyle program that helped him achieve greater fitness, lower cholesterol, lower blood pressure, and have the energy and strength of someone half his age. In this book, he shares what he learned from his own experiences.

During the last decade, it's become increasingly clear that no matter how good our technology becomes—drugs and devices—the root causes of most of the chronic diseases in this country are primarily related to the diet and lifestyle choices we make each day. These include what we eat, how we respond to stress, whether or not we smoke, how much we exercise (and, as emphasized in this book, how we exercise), and how much love and support we have in our lives.

In our research during the past thirty-five years, my colleagues and I at the non-profit Preventive Medicine Research Institute found that when we address these root causes of our health and well-being, our bodies often have a remarkable capacity to begin healing, and much more quickly than had once been thought possible.

This book is timely. As you know, the obesity epidemic is real. If you want to see something really scary, go to the web site of the Centers for Disease Control and Prevention in Atlanta, which has been tracking the rise in obesity (http://www.cdc.gov/nccdphp/dnpa/obesity/trend/maps/). You can see the obesity epidemic spreading like cancer metastasizing across the country from 1985 until now. It looks like an alien force or a conquering army is taking over the U.S., state-by-state, year-by-year.

Almost two-thirds of adults are overweight, one-third of whom are obese. Even worse, a study in the Annals of Internal Medicine that followed 4,000 people over 30 years found that 9 out of 10 men and 7 out of 10 women will eventually become overweight if current trends continue.

According to the U.S. Department of Health and Human Services, obesity may account for 300,000 deaths a year, almost as many as deaths from cigarette smoking. People who are obese have a 50-100 percent increased risk of premature death from all causes—including heart disease, diabetes, high blood pressure, gallbladder disease, sleep apnea, osteoarthritis and some cancers—compared to those who are not overweight.

And it's not just adults. This may be the first generation in which kids live a shorter lifespan than their parents. Since 1970, the percentage of kids who are overweight or obese has risen almost fourfold, from 4.2 percent to 15.3 percent. According to former Surgeon General Richard Carmona, M.D., "As we look to the future and where childhood obesity will be in 20 years…it is every bit as threatening to us as is the terrorist threat we face today. It is the threat from within."

Well, it doesn't have to be this way. We can do better. We can have a significant impact on our personal health and our children's health by taking care of ourselves, one person at a time. The chapter in Tim's book describing how he teaches children about fitness and eating is particularly helpful in addressing the current obesity crisis. The best teacher for your kids is being a good example for them.

Over 75% of the $2.8 trillion in health care costs are due to chronic diseases. Heart disease and type 2 diabetes, which account for more deaths in the U.S. and worldwide than everything else combined, are nearly completely preventable by making comprehensive lifestyle changes. Today. We don't need to wait for a new drug or laser or high-tech breakthrough; we simply need to put into practice the ideas described in this book.

We can make much better health care available for many more people at far lower costs when we change the underlying lifestyle causes of disease rather than only treating the disease after the development of symptoms—and the only side-effects are good ones.

In addition to preventing chronic diseases, these comprehensive lifestyle changes may often reverse the progression of these illnesses, as I discuss in Chapter 5 of this book. At a time when the power of comprehensive lifestyle changes to prevent and reverse chronic diseases is becoming clearly documented, the limitations and costs of high-tech medicine are also becoming increasingly clear. The latest studies show that comprehensive lifestyle changes often work even better than drugs and surgery in treating many chronic diseases.

For example, a series of randomized controlled trials have shown that angioplasties and stents do not prolong life or prevent heart attacks in stable patients. Only 1 out of 49 men who undergoes surgery or radiation for prostate cancer lives longer; the others often become impotent or incontinent, or both. Up to one-half of Americans are projected to be diabetic or pre-diabetic in the next eight years, but lifestyle changes work better than drugs at preventing and treating the complications of type 2 diabetes at a fraction of the costs.

It's not all or nothing. In our research, we found that the more you change your diet and lifestyle, the more you're likely to improve. At any age. What matters most is your overall way of eating and living. If you indulge yourself one day, eat healthier the next. If you don't have time to exercise or meditate one day, do a little more the next. You get the idea.

In our research, we also found that when you change your lifestyle, you change your genes—"turning on" hundreds of genes that keep you healthy, and "turning off" hundreds of genes that promote heart disease, type 2 diabetes, breast cancer, prostate cancer, and other chronic diseases in only three months. Our genes are a predisposition, but our genes are not our fate. We have more control over our health and well-being than many people realize.

So, your health is clearly much more in your control than you may have once believed. This is one of the key messages in Tim's book—not to blame, but to empower. With even a modest time commitment and following some basic and mostly common sense guidelines about what you eat and how you approach exercise, you're likely to make a meaningful impact on your metabolism, weight, strength and well-being.

In this innovative book, Tim has helped to pinpoint some of the root causes of the obesity epidemic. He's provided some very specific and sustainable approaches to help adults get thinner, fitter, and healthier. The importance of finding "teachable, learnable and sustainable" methods to deal with weight, fitness and youthfulness has never been greater. I hope that readers of this book will follow the methods and teaching in it to enjoy a long and healthy life.

WWW.ORNISH.COM

❧ *Reader Reviews* ❧

Excellent book, way more worth than it is priced!

"This book is the only book on OBESITY that clearly explains not only the epidemic and its cause but also how to effectively lose weight and keep it off. Once I started reading I did not put it down until I was done. It is very simple reading and the author has explained everything in detail. The information he provides is based on scientific studies and peer review literature. You do not need another book to lose weight if you have this one. Excellent buy."

Amazon.com

Solid research.

"At long last: Solid research from a real authority that can help countless change their lives."

Amazon.com

Finally, a sensible and effective book on weight loss.

Burn Calories While You Sleep is a catchy title, but even more importantly gives the reader an orderly and fully explained method to lose weight. When to eat and when to stop-simple intelligence! The exercises require as little time as the author claims and are effective. Dr. Fischell's writing method is easy to read and humorous and does not leave the reader with any ambiguous ideas. This little book alone could reverse the obesity epidemic in the US. I hope that those that need it will buy it and I am sure they won't be disappointed!"

Amazon.com

Lots of helpful gems.

"I like Burn Calories While You Sleep, and found it useful for several reasons:

Burn Calories contains lots of helpful gems. I have watched my diet and exercised faithfully since college, so I'm reasonably fit. However, as the author mentions, the fight is becoming a little more difficult as I approach middle-age. After reading this book I've realized I can incorporate a few additional simple strategies into my routine to maintain my fitness level as I age.

The advice in Burn Calories can be applied "on the road." I travel frequently for work and fun, which presents some challenges to staying fit: long hours in confined spaces, inadequate exercise facilities and reliance on restaurants. With seated crunches and isometric fidgeting (chapter three) I can exercise while I fly/drive. The majority of the recommended exercises can be performed in a hotel room with the aid of resistance bands, which are light and fit into a suitcase. The author offers dietary rules rather than a diet that can be applied anywhere.

Burn Calories is readable. The author writes in his own voice (and he includes some humor), which makes for much more enjoyable reading than dry how-to tomes. In addition, it's concise: no fluff here. I read it from cover-to-cover on a flight.

It makes sense. The author includes the "why" behind his methodologies. And, the information is organized logically: the main points are outlined at the end of each chapter."

Amazon.com

I recommend.

"Burn Calories While You Sleep: I discovered plenty of helpful gems in it that I was able to adopt effortlessly without changing my lifestyle."

Amazon.com

A great read!

"This is an incredibly well-written guide on a very important issue that will be helpful and relevant to anyone!"

Amazon.com

A common sense approach.

"Here is a common sense approach that anyone can follow to finally tackle one of the top health issues of our time. No more fading fads du jour. Follow Dr. Fischell's new reset rules and reap a lifetime of health and well-being."

Amazon.com

I highly recommend this book.

"I consider myself to be a very health conscience person. Even though weight problem is not my top concern, I still find this book very worthwhile. What the book offers is a very comprehensive yet practical approach to a healthy way of living. I find myself being educated on many levels: understanding diet and food; understanding my body and its metabolism; understanding the effects of different types of exercises. I am the sort of person who always likes to know the reasons behind the practices. In other words, if I am doing something, I know why I am doing it. This book gives me many answers to my questions. I highly recommend this book to my friends and anybody who values health and quality of life more than anything else."

Amazon.com

Recommend this program!

"This book gives some very practical ways to tone your body...even with driving, (while not texting) quick, easy, and good summaries. Would recommend this program! And if you can't afford weights, use milk jugs filled with H2O at your level."

Amazon.com

Simple and sensible book on weight loss.

"Well written and thought fully explained; simple steps in daily routine that helps in maintaining weight and also helps to lose weight."

Amazon.com

This book will help you if you are serious about losing weight.

"This is a book for people who want to lose weight and keep it off. For people who truly want to improve their health, not just shed pounds for an upcoming event. Dr. Fischell has boiled down decades of research into a few rules for people who are serious about making changes to their lifestyle. It will only work if you put in the effort, but the payoff is huge."

David J. Maron, MD
Professor of Medicine and Emergency Medicine
Vanderbilt University Medical Center
Medical Director, Vanderbilt Dayani Center for Health and Wellness

"You can't help getting older,
but you don't have to get old."
George Burns

"It's not the years in your life that count,
it's the life in your years."
Abraham Lincoln

❧ Table of Contents ❧

✌ *Introduction* ✌

Nearly 70% of American's are overweight or obese. We are inundated with statistics, news stories, TV shows, documentaries, magazine articles, books and infomercials about the obesity epidemic, and for good reason. The problems related to overeating and under-metabolizing what we eat are enormous. The toll on our joints, our hearts, our health care system, and our self-esteem are enormous.

This is now not just a national and now a worldwide epidemic. Obesity and the related morbidity and mortality is one of the leading causes of the healthcare crisis in the United States. If nothing changes in our society, it is expected that the obesity rate will climb to 42% of the U.S. population by 2030. It is predicted that the number of Americans that are "severely obese" (i.e., more than 100 pounds overweight) will also double, to 11% of the population in the next 20 years. Forget about "Obamacare," and other healthcare related budget crises. If we could just stabilize the obesity epidemic it is predicted that this would save $550 billion in healthcare costs over the next 20 years. What are we going to do about this?

There has been a lot written to try to help people fight this challenging health issue. Shortly after starting this book I walked into the health and fitness section of Barnes and Noble to see what others had written in the field. I was shocked and overwhelmed by the sheer number of books about dieting, nutrition, weight lifting, exercising, being thin, etc. My first reaction was, wow, maybe there is no need for another book teaching about fitness and weight loss. It has all been said before! But then, I looked around the store and saw what you see every day on the streets and in the malls of America. Overweight adults. A lot of them. This group is growing in girth, and in numbers as a percentage of our population every month, every year. Obviously none of these books are resonating with people. There is no movement. These books are four-hundred pages long, and filled with so much detailed information and psychobabble that much of the valuable and sustainable messaging in them is lost. America is not reading, listening or acting. The messages are too detailed or too vague and are lost in translation.

So what is this book about and why is it different from the hundreds of other books that are have been written in the last decade to address this issue? First of all, this book is based on science, not beliefs, hype and marketing. Everything in this book is referenced to human physiology and real science, published in articles in peer reviewed medical journals. You will not be given some robotic workout routine, or a thirty-page list of healthy foods.

4

You will learn why human beings gain weight as they get older, and conversely, how you can sustainably maintain or lose weight. When you understand how the human body works with regard to the conversion of food to energy (or fat) and how energy is burned (i.e., metabolism), you will be more motivated to change your behaviors to take advantage of this knowledge. As Descartes said, "Knowledge is power."

This is not a fad book. It is a common sense book. There will be no recommendations about trendy new diets based on grapefruits or oxtails, untested herbal remedies, complex recipes, or ridiculous exercise programs that Hercules himself would struggle with. This is also not a thirty-day fitness plan, or a make a better butt book. It is a lifelong and sustainable fitness plan. This book is about the rest of your life, not about fitting into a dress for a wedding next month.

Most importantly, in this era of time pressure, the program and lifestyle changes outlined in this book will not require you to spend 25% of your conscious life trying to follow complex instructions, counting calories, day-by-day detailed punch lists of what to eat, or the specific list of exercises in a "daily" workout. The path is relatively simple and highly efficient. I want 40 minutes of your time 2-3 times per week. If you do this, and you can, you will be pleased if not shocked at what you can achieve.

Think about this. You are only given one body. Your body and its health, strength and well-being is the most valuable possession you will ever have. Most people care more about their dog or their new flat panel TV than they do about their body and their health. It is time to give your body and your physical being the respect, attention, love and care that it deserves. The dividends for taking care of your temple (your body) are huge.

The main focus of this book is to provide a set of rules or guidelines that can be imprinted in your brain to allow you to become thin (or at least thinner), fit and energized, and feeling young (or younger). Of course, one cannot achieve this without some pain (that is the 40 minutes 2-3 times per week), and without some changes to dietary behavior. Two plus two does equal four. If you eat more than you burn you will gain weight. If you burn more than you eat you will lose weight. This ties in to the first specific advice to readers of the book.

Some people just like to eat (a lot) and are unable or unwilling to make even modest changes in their eating behavior. So, if you are an individual who eats 6,000-7,000 calories a day and cannot, or will not change this behavior, or if you think that this book is about burning calories with some electrical appliance attached to your bed, I will give an important piece of advice. Sell this book to a friend. I cannot help you.

For the rest of you, who are motivated, and willing to listen, you will learn a lot from this book. You will learn why we tend to gain weight as we get older, and how to reverse this, change your metabolic rate, and literally burn calories while you sleep. You will learn why walking on a treadmill for an hour and a half, six days a week will not solve your weight problem. You will realize why fad diets and fad exercising do not work. You will also learn other incredible and simple pearls and tips about raising healthy and fit children, living longer, and staying young as you age. I also promise to keep the book short and sweet. I know you are very busy. This will not be a four-hundred-page treatise, but a concise outline to achieve a healthier and more youthful future for you and your children. It is teachable, learnable and sustainable.

❧ Chapter One ❧

AGING AND METABOLISM: YES. IT'S TRUE. YOU ARE EATING LESS AND GAINING WEIGHT

It is very common. The nurse in the office weighs my patient and records his height and weight. The patient is a 58 year-old man who is 5' 9" tall and weighs 256 pounds. One year ago at his office visit he weighed 243 pounds. We talk about it. I explain to him that his increasing weight is a major health issue. It is causing high blood pressure, and a slightly elevated blood glucose level. This is either early type 2 diabetes or at the very least the metabolic syndrome (pre-diabetes). These two risk factors, diabetes and hypertension, combined with his sedentary lifestyle, poor eating habits and an elevated cholesterol level, despite medications, will lead to a high risk of heart attack or stroke in the next ten years. There are other tolls related to his obesity that will eventually disable or kill him over the next twenty years.

Even this moderate level of obesity will have consequences of low energy and fatigue from the work of carrying that much extra weight around every day. I try to put this into perspective for him. I am 6' and 160 pounds. I tell him to imagine how exhausted I would be at the end of each day if someone forced me to wear a backpack with 100 lbs. of lead weights in it, and walk all day with this on my back. I can assure you that even though I am fit, I would collapse from exhaustion by nightfall. That is exactly what my patient is doing. He is carrying an extra 100 lbs. of weight around with him, all day, every day.

I tell him he should exercise regularly. He tells me he is too tired and too busy, and besides, he tried the treadmill thing and it really did not work for him. I tell him that he needs to eat healthier, and less. He then says, "But you know Doc, I am eating less than I did when I was 30 years old and I keep gaining weight." And you know what I tell him? "You are right"! This is a nearly universal observation among both men and women as they age, especially adults in their 40s, 50s and 60s. It is real. It is related to a predictable drop in metabolic rate as sedentary adults age. What is happening?

Changes in Metabolic Rate with Age

The patient above is not at all unusual. He is just like millions of men and women in America and in other "modernized" countries. It creeps up on them. He was not always overweight. Over the last twenty-five years his waist size has crept up from 32" at age 25, to 34" at age 35, to 37" at age 45, and now close to a 39"

9

waist at age 58. This is not far from the average change in waist size in American men, as tracked over the last decade. The average American male in 2011 has a waist size of 40". This is a lot of new fat being stored as abdominal fat, which is a major, independent predictor of heart attack risk.

So, if he (or she) is eating less than he was at age 30 and he is gaining weight, what is the change that has caused this? This is the critical question to ask if one hopes to reverse this unhealthy trend. Remember, "two plus two equals four." If you are eating less and gaining weight there must be a fundamental change in how many calories you are burning each day. Yes, he is less active physically than when he was 35 years old. However, this only accounts for a relatively small proportion of the imbalance. The major shift in the formula is due to a fundamental, age-related change in basal (resting, day-to-day) metabolic rate (BMR). What is the cause of this loss of metabolic rate as we age? I have asked more than six-hundred people this question and virtually *no one*, including dozens of M.D.s, knew the answer to this question. Critically, *if you don't know the answer to this question then you cannot know the solution to the problem*!

This change in metabolic rate is caused predominantly by a measurable and often profound change in skeletal muscle (lean) body mass, which occurs in unfit adults with aging. In addition, there is an important and additive change due to a decrease in the metabolic activity of the skeletal muscle that you have left.

This message about metabolic rate and its relationship to the amount and metabolic activity of your skeletal muscle is critical. In most adults, skeletal muscle accounts for approximately 70% of all the calories that we burn each day. Skeletal muscle is the fuel burning system for your body. If one looks at skeletal muscle mass (biceps, triceps, quadriceps, gluteus, abdominal, lower back, pectoral, etc.) over time there is a substantial decline in muscle mass from age 20 to 60 in most adults (see Figure 1). Not only do most Americans have much less muscle at age 60 than at age 20 or 30, but the muscle we have is not being used very much. It has become metabolically dormant. It is not being "stressed" with exercise.

When muscle fibers are not "stressed" they will atrophy (get smaller) and lose their thirst for glucose, the main metabolic "fuel" molecule. In untrained muscle of sedentary adults there is a profound loss of mitochondria in the muscle cells. These mitochondria are critical in turning glucose plus oxygen into energy. Old, and sedentary skeletal muscles are weak and do not use much energy at rest, which also can profoundly reduce "metabolic rate" both at rest and during physical activity. The loss of muscle and muscle strength due to aging and a sedentary lifestyle also has a profound effect on day-to-day life and physical function, and will also shorten life expectancy.

The result of this "double hit" of, 1) loss of muscle, and 2) loss of the metabolic (glucose burning) demands and capability of the muscle that we have left can lead to dramatic changes in our basal metabolic rate, and our strength, as we age. Most relatively sedentary adults will drop their day-to-day metabolic burn rate by 30-50% between age 20 and age 60. This is why we can eat less than we did when we were young and continuously gain weight. How can this trend be reversed? Can we alter our metabolic rate as we age and burn calories like a twenty-five-year-old again? The answer is "Yes!"

In the next chapter we will outline, and define a game-plan to rebuild skeletal muscle mass, regain fit, trained, and actively metabolizing, and strong, skeletal muscle, and reverse this downward spiral of eating less, gaining weight, being less active, that plagues so many adults. We will teach you how to dramatically increase your metabolic rate, eat well (and less), feel energized, and lose weight. You will also become physically much stronger. You will be able to carry out the physical activities of daily life with less effort and with better balance and poise.

A Primer in Metabolism: What Do We Burn? How Do We Gain Weight? How Do We Lose Weight?

I am going to try to keep this simple. I apologize to the nutritional physiologists who could easily write a three-hundred-page book about human metabolism. This is the (very) short version.

If you want to lose weight, it is important to understand some fundamental, and to some extent, common sense principals about losing weight despite the aging process. It is important to understand how the body deals with food intake, and how and why it uses excess food intake to create stored energy, mostly in the form of fat.

Excess food is ultimately stored in the form of glycogen (a complex carbohydrate stored in our muscles and liver) and fat (adipose tissue) in order to supply the energy needed to meet the body's metabolic demands when food is not plentiful.

This storing of excess food as fat and then burning it later when food was not around was critical to survival in primitive man. Human existence, for millions of years, was truly feast or famine. If you could not store excess calories as fat during feasts, you would literally starve to death during famines. So this storing of excess food as fat was, evolutionarily, highly adaptive for our primitive ancestors. Unfortunately, it is highly destructive in modern cultures, when food is available all the time, and in super-size quantities. When we combine this modern bounty of food, combined with a sedentary lifestyle, you get a society (like America) where 2/3 of the adults are overweight or obese.

FOOD AND METABOLISM: THE BASICS

Glucose is a very simple sugar molecule (monosacharride). It is the basic unit of energy supply to cells in the human body. Glucose combined with oxygen allows your cells to make ATP (adenosine triphosphate). When the phosphate molecule of ATP is broken off in the cell, energy is released. It is this chain of glucose plus oxygen, creating ATP that creates energy from the burning of glucose, very much like gasoline used to fuel the internal combustion engine of a car. Much of this takes place in the mitochondria inside the cell.

Ultimately, all food, or stored fat, must be converted into glucose, or other small molecules, like acetyl CoA in order to supply energy to our cells. When we eat, the food is absorbed in the small intestine. Very simple foods like table sugar (sucrose, a disaccharide) and simple processed starches are converted to glucose and can quickly increase blood glucose levels. More complex carbohydrates, like the ones contained in most fresh fruits and vegetables are converted more slowly into glucose. Proteins take even more time and energy in the intestines and the liver to be converted into its component amino acids (protein building blocks). Amino acids can then be converted into glucose, when other fuel sources are scarce. Thus, proteins take a relatively long time, through complex and energy consuming steps to be converted into glucose. Proteins and amino acids will also be used to build or re-build stressed muscle fibers when we stress our skeletal muscle, and may not be converted to glucose at all. This is important to remember when we talk about why eating protein is a key to muscle building and remodeling, and to losing weight. Atkins was right.

How about fats in our diet? When we eat fatty foods it is really bad. Fats are absorbed rather quickly, converted to various fat molecules, like triglycerides, and then shipped off to organs, mainly fat cells (adipocytes) to be stored as fat. This process of rapid fat absorption and storage, and the conversion of glucose to fat is driven by the key hormone insulin, which is secreted by beta-cells in the pancreas.

Diabetes and Obesity: A Huge and Growing Problem (no pun intended)

The obesity epidemic in America and other western cultures is perhaps the biggest healthcare crisis today. It is the

15

predominant cause of the explosion in type 2 (adult onset) diabetes. In a recent USA Today article, they note that 14% of Americans are diabetic. Even more frighteningly, experts predict that this may soar to close to 40% of the population by 2050!

Diabetes is the number one cause of kidney failure, adult blindness, limb amputation, and a huge contributor to coronary artery disease and stroke. It is an accelerator of atherosclerosis causing plaque buildup in our arteries throughout our body. The Center for Disease Control (CDC) estimates that diabetes currently costs the U.S. $174 billion per year, most of which is in direct healthcare costs. The cost, like the incidence, may nearly triple in the next 40 years to $500 billion per year if we do not stop this alarming explosion in obesity!

How do we become diabetic? Insulin is the bad actor! Rapid insulin release or insulin spikes occur in response to a significant and rapid increase in our blood glucose level. So, when we eat sweets (high sugar and processed carbohydrate content), or a huge meal of any type, our insulin levels rise quickly and dramatically. A high glucose level is the signal to our body that there is excessive food in our life. The message is, "Wow, food is plentiful, feast time, let's store it as fat!" In very overweight adults who eat a lot, the pancreas works overtime and keeps producing a lot of insulin. This extra insulin in your blood will add to the problem, and make you even fatter. The body eventually makes fewer insulin receptors on the cell surface so we become "insulin resistant," and glucose is not metabolized as quickly into glycogen and fat. Eventually we become so resistant to the effects of insulin that we cannot store the glucose in our body fast enough and our blood glucose levels are elevated, even when we are not eating! This is type 2 diabetes.

This is not just a huge problem for society and our overburdened healthcare system. It is really harmful to you as an individual. Diabetes will triple the risk of heart attack and stroke, more than double the risk of developing kidney failure and blindness, triple the risk of developing peripheral neuropathy, and recently has been found to also nearly double the risk of developing Alzheimer's dementia. The prognosis and effect on life expectancy from this condition is about the same as breast cancer or colon cancer. This is a disabling and deadly disease.

Here is the exciting news. Diabetes is nearly totally preventable and even curable! The main difference between type 2 diabetes in an overweight adult and cancer is that you do not need surgery, radiation or chemotherapy to cure your "cancer" (i.e., the diabetes). If you lose 50-100 pounds—depending on how overweight you are—you can prevent this condition. If you already have diabetes, you can lose weight and cure your diabetes. Let's think about this. If you had colon or breast cancer, and I told you that you could cure your cancer by losing 75 pounds, would you do it? I think we both know the answer. The cure is in your hands. Read this book, follow the guidelines, prevent or cure your diabetes and live much longer.

Why Bother? I Am Not Diabetic. It Is Too Much Work, and What Are the Problems With Being Overweight?

There is no question. Humans are resistant to change. This is especially true if they do not see immediate positive reinforcement. It is always easier to just go back to your "usual" dietary and sedentary habits. Even though the behavioral changes outlined in this book are pretty simple and will work for just about everyone, this will not happen in thirty days. Be patient and know that if you follow the major key points in this book, week in and week out you will have a huge impact on your life. We are talking 20-50 years! You will be able to lose weight and achieve close to your ideal body weight, and without a huge time commitment. But why do it?

There are numerous and serious consequences to not doing this (i.e., staying 50-150 lbs. overweight). What will you gain by becoming fit and getting closer to your ideal body weight? A lot.

18

You will have much more energy, stamina and physical strength. It will improve your mood (less depressed). You will reduce your blood pressure and possibly eliminate the need for blood pressure medications. You will substantially decrease your risk of a heart attack or stroke, and prevent the onset of type 2 diabetes. You will reduce cancer risks. You will reduce the likelihood and/or delay severe osteoarthritis of your knees and hips that may eventually disable you or require hip or knee replacement. You will double or triple your muscle and core strength which will allow you to participate in an active life, including tennis, basketball, racket sports, biking, hiking, dancing, skiing, etc., well into your 70s. You will reduce the likelihood of a ruptured disc in your back. If you are a woman, and adopt this fitness routine you will slow or reverse osteoporosis. You will look better and be more attractive to your spouse, boyfriend or girlfriend. You will fit better in those horrible coach seats on airplanes. You can play touch football with the kids, or grandkids. You will look forward to wearing a bathing suit at the beach. You will have better (and probably more) sex! You will have enhanced self-esteem and self-confidence. You are more likely to get that job you interviewed for. You will (statistically) live five-to-ten years longer. If that is not enough to motivate you, then you should give this book to a friend.

CHAPTER ONE KEY POINTS: METABOLISM

1) Metabolic rate falls dramatically with aging in sedentary adults.

2) Loss of skeletal muscle mass and inactive muscles is main cause of 1). This also make you weak.

3) Insulin is the main hormone instructing our body to store food as fat.

4) Overeating (big meals) and carbohydrates raise insulin levels.

5) Carbohydrates and sugar rapidly raise glucose and get stored as fat.

6) Ingested fat gets processed quickly, and is stored as fat.

7) As you get obese you make a lot of insulin, which stores even more fat.

8) Obesity creates type 2 diabetes, a common and fatal disease.

9) Type 2 diabetes is preventable or curable by losing weight.

10) Obesity carries a huge price tag. It is not really "OK."

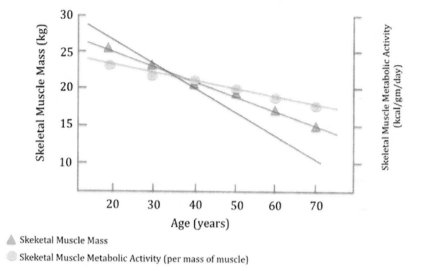

Figure 1

AGING AND METABOLISM:

Closely related to the mass and metabolism of your skeletal muscle. This is a graph showing the predicted loss of muscle mass in sedentary adults as they age (line with triangles), and the predicted loss of resting metabolic activity (glucose burned per day for each kilogram of remaining muscle) with age (line with circles). When one combines the loss of muscle mass with the loss of muscle metabolic activity you get an even more profound drop in resting metabolic rate with aging in sedentary adults (straight line).

❧ *Chapter Two* ❦

Change Your Metabolic Rate and Burn Calories While You Sleep Weight Lifting (Not Body Building): You Can Do This!

I once had the privilege of playing a memorable round of golf at Augusta National Golf Club with the great college football coach, Lou Holtz. After a short time it became clear why "Coach" Holtz has been so successful in his professional life (and he is thin and fit to boot). Before we arrived at Augusta National Golf Club, he informed us that, "These are the rules!" He went on to bark out a list of key rules for his guests at the golf course. These were not offered as optional. These Rules were not just to be followed if you felt like it. These were the "RULES!"

I am going to start this chapter telling you that this pretty simple and highly efficient fitness and weight loss program will work if you remember every day, "These are the Rules." There are not hundreds of rules. There are about ten rules or "Key Points" for each of the first five "Key" chapters. Not too bad. 40-50 key points to incorporate into your behavior in order to transform your life.

If your attention span and memory do not allow you to immediately learn and imprint these rules in your conscious and subconscious mind, I suggest that you make the copies of the Key points or Rules from each of these critical chapters and tape them on your refrigerator (especially the rules for eating). Read them every morning until they are imbedded in your brain, no less than your basic sense of values, your route to work, or the names of your children. When you do, you will succeed.

These messages become even more powerful when you teach them and verbalize them to your friends and loved ones. Indeed, the most powerful way to learn the rules is to share and teach them, just like remembering a joke by retelling it several times. Your loved ones and co-workers will get it, and so will you! The rules are not rocket science. They make a lot of sense. They are often just "common sense." Some are even pretty funny. You have heard many of them before but probably have not organized them or consistently incorporated them into your behavioral value system. If you share, and live these rules with your friends and loved ones, then we all can work together to begin to change the culture of obesity. A pass it forward mentality!

ENOUGH WITH THE PEP TALK! WHAT SHOULD I DO?

You knew it was coming. This is the pain part. Trust me, this is not so bad, and much less annoying than being bored for two hours on a treadmill, five days a week (see Chapter Four). Unlike some mind-boggling fad thirty-day-workout plans, this is also a fitness routine that can be started to match your current level of conditioning, and then built upon over time by ordinary, unfit and overweight adults. You do not have to be a world-class athlete or even that coordinated to do these exercises. You can do this!

Aerobic weight lifting, with circuit training, to be described shortly, is the key to efficiently altering your metabolic rate and reversing the downward spiral of losing actively metabolizing skeletal muscle. We have to re-build skeletal muscle in your body and make it metabolically active and trained young skeletal muscle. The most efficient way to achieve this is by lifting weights.

Many people equate lifting weights with body building. This is not the goal. The Burn Calories workout plan will not make you look like Arnold Schwarzenegger in his prime, or a contestant in a bodybuilding contest. However, after as little as two-to-three months you will be amazed at how much better you look. You will begin to have muscle definition (i.e., the ability to see the outline of your muscles) under a thinner layer of fat. You will get positive feedback, in the mirror, from friends and loved ones, and on the bathroom scale. The goal is to rebuild lean, not bulky, strong and actively metabolizing skeletal muscle. Eventually, even if you get to thin you will be strong.

WEIGHT LIFTING FOR BODY BUILDING (BAD) VS. "AEROBIC" WEIGHT TRAINING TO BUILD LEAN, FIT AND METABOLICALLY ACTIVE MUSCLE (GOOD)!

The key difference between building lean and mean, and actively metabolizing skeletal muscle and building large and bulky muscles is related to the amount of weight you are lifting, and the number of reps or repetitions of the muscle exercise with a given amount of weight. If you lift as much as you can lift for three-to-four reps, this will build bulky, body-builder muscles. This is also, in my opinion, not very healthy. Heavy weight lifting will put severe stress on your joints (shoulders, knees, hips, etc.) and can cause immediate and/or long-term damage.

When you lift very heavy weights you have to bear down hard in order to stabilize your back and avoid a ruptured disc, or other joint damage. In medicine this bearing down is called a valsalva maneuver. Have you seen the look on the weightlifters' faces at the Olympics? It looks like their eyes are almost popping

25

out of their heads. This is not healthy. When you bear down that hard, it rapidly and dramatically increases your blood pressure. This sudden explosion in blood pressure may even promote a rupture of a plaque in a heart artery. This could start a heart attack. One could even rupture an aneurysm in a brain blood vessel and cause a stroke. Even though these risks are low, it is not a great exercise plan. In addition it is too hard, and it will not achieve the goals set forth in this book. It will make you look bulky. This is not the look most women are looking for. It may also make you gain weight rather than lose weight. Just like hours on a treadmill, this is not the ticket!

We are going to pursue a little bit kinder and gentler approach to our workout. If you do repeated stressful weight lifting of moderate weights, particularly in an aerobic method, with very little rest between sets of lifting, as taught in this book, you will build lean and larger, but not large, metabolically active skeletal muscle. Even though you will not be lifting heavy weights in this method, don't be fooled about the intention or the effect. This weight training is short duration, moderate weight, but HIGH intensity. Without the high intensity component of the workout, you will not transform your skeletal muscle and change your metabolism. It is this creation, and constant remodeling of stressed skeletal muscle mass that burns calories and increases your metabolic rate. We want to stress the muscles hard, but without heavy weight lifting. This workout is focused on short duration, moderate weight, high intensity, "aerobic" weight lifting!

The Anti-Aging Effects of Weight-Based Stressing of Skeletal Muscle

There is another incredible benefit to the type of stress on skeletal muscle fibers that is created by the exercise program outlined in this book. Anti-aging! I am not necessarily talking about the extra six-to-seven years that lean and fit adults add to their life expectancy compared to sedentary adults. This is well established.

I am referring to research that has focused upon the cellular effects of aging in skeletal muscle in humans. As we have already discussed, sedentary adults lose a lot of skeletal muscle mass with age. Perhaps even more interesting, and relevant, is the observation that the muscle that is left in these sedentary adults looks very different at age 50 or 60 than it did at age 20.

As sedentary adults age, one sees a significant change in the appearance of the skeletal muscle cell under a microscope. Biopsies from sedentary, middle-aged adults, reveals that the untrained muscle looks old. These muscle cells are atrophied and smaller, with less muscle fibers and with less contractile protein (actin and myosin). More importantly, the cells have very few

27

mitochondria compared to a young person's muscle. Mitochondria are the tiny, sub-cellular structures that take oxygen and glucose, and generate the energy in the muscle cell that is needed for cell metabolism and for muscle contraction.

Skeletal muscle cells with fewer, and perhaps less functional, mitochondria will not be able to generate as much force, will get fatigued more quickly, and will burn fewer calories during work and at rest. This is one of the main reasons why you are weaker, fatter and fatigue more easily with physical activity than when you were twenty-five years old. This is why you see your father or grandmother wobble and nearly fall when they get out of a chair. They are weak. The other fascinating and important observation is that this cellular aging effect and the loss of mitochondria can be prevented or reversed by stressing the muscle with weight lifting, especially when done as outlined in this book.

In one very interesting study by Little, and his colleagues, they found profound changes in human skeletal muscle cells with short duration (20 minutes per session) high intensity skeletal muscle stress done three times per week for only two weeks. In trained and stressed muscle of older adults the number of mitochondria increase, and the muscle begins to look like young skeletal muscle again. Other significant metabolic changes are observed that would be associated with greater muscle strength and endurance. Thus, short duration, high intensity muscle stress is a key stimulus for anti-aging adaptations of our skeletal muscle. The aging of muscle can be reversed with weight lifting and stressful (high intensity) exercise. Adults can rebuild skeletal muscle cells that look young, with more mitochondria, and a greater ability to contract, and burn calories. In the next chapter, we will focus on the type of workout that can efficiently help you to rebuild muscle, strength and metabolic activity, and turn back the clock. After a few years of keeping with this you may be able to boast, as I do, that I am at my high school graduation weight, but twice as strong as I was when I was twenty years old. What a great goal. It is achievable.

CHAPTER TWO KEY POINTS: CHANGING YOUR METABOLIC RATE

1) Change your health you must embrace new "Rules."

2) Skeletal muscle burns ~ 70% of calories burned every day.

3) Old and untrained skeletal muscle cells lose mitochondria (tiny energy generators), are weak and metabolically sluggish.

4) To increase metabolic rate you must build new skeletal muscle.

5) Heavy weight lifting (body building) is hard, and may not be healthy.

6) Building and maintaining (stressed) skeletal muscle burns calories.

7) Aerobic (high intensity) weight lifting to stress skeletal muscle will reverse the cellular changes, increase mitochondria, make muscle stronger and metabolically active and make YOU strong, fit and thin, efficiently!

❧ *Chapter Three* ❦

The "Burn Calories" Workout

Getting Started: Setting Your Workout Routine and Making It Bearable (maybe even fun)

Before we start the actual workout, we need to outline some key points to make this routine sustainable, and even enjoyable. First, you need to decide when to do your workouts. Some people, like me, are morning people. That is when I have the most energy. I also find that doing a workout early, and before I go to work, gets me energized for the rest of the day and eliminates working out as a chore on my to-do list for later that day.

Other people just cannot get started in the morning, or have to take the kids to school, etc. You can do this in the afternoon or evening. The important thing to do is to pick the days and the times that work for you, and to stick with it. It is sometimes more fun and motivating if you can do this with a friend or spouse, or a personal trainer, if you can afford it. If you make an appointment with someone else for this time, it is harder to just skip it. As you will learn, however, the Burn Calories workout is not really a social event. It is a focused, high intensity, but short duration, aerobic, workout. If you do this workout properly you will not have the time, or energy to discuss the gubernatorial race, or the latest movie review during the workout. You will be breathing pretty hard for the 20-25 minutes that you are lifting weights.

You need to do this workout at least every third day. Ideally, you will do this workout three or four times per week when you are starting out, especially if you are trying lose weight, and not just maintain your achieved ideal weight goal from being fit. It is not necessary or very helpful to do this every day. Your muscles need time to recover and remodel for 36-48 hours after this workout. That is when you are burning calories as you sleep. After you have changed your metabolic rate, lost the weight and have become fit, and you are following the eating rules in Chapter Five, you may be able to maintain your weight and fitness with as little as two workouts per week. Eventually, this will become ingrained in your life's routine and you will not want to ever miss your workout.

Finally, one tip that may get you energized and pumped up at seven in the morning. Music! This works for me, and many others. Get the tiny iPod Shuffle ($49) or its equivalent. Load about 100-200 of your favorite workout songs. It does not matter whether it's jazz or techno dance, or rock and roll. Buy a decent pair of ear buds ($25-$75). If you can afford it, spend a little more, and get some Shure or Monster (or inexpensive) ear buds. Start the music. Crank it up, and start your workout. If you would rather listen to an audio-book, or to silence, that is fine too. You can decide what works for you.

The Aerobic "Warm-Up"

You will begin every workout with a 10-15-minute aerobic "warm-up". If you really love this type of activity you can do this for more than 15 minutes. However, spending 30-60 minutes here is not critical to the success of the mission of changing your metabolic rate. It is not part of the "time-efficient" workout focus taught in this book (see Chapter Four). There should be no excuses. You do not need to belong to a gym to do this workout. At the end of the chapter we will discuss what little home exercise equipment you will need to do this workout for the readers who do not have access to a health club.

You can choose what you like to do for the aerobic warm-up phase. For many people, an elliptical machine is a great low impact warm-up option. This is a particularly good warm-up if you use an elliptical machine that incorporates the arms and upper body. It is good to get as many muscle groups as possible engaged in this warm-up phase of the workout. There are many other options if you do not have access to a gym or an elliptical machine. Other options for the aerobic 15-minute warm-up would include stationary bicycle (or real cycling), a treadmill (or walking/jogging), rowing machine, stair climber machine (or climbing stairs), swimming, dancing, Pilates, kick boxing, basketball, or any other aerobic activity that uses most of your muscles and gets your heart rate elevated. The goal is to get your muscles and you heart and lungs "warmed-up" for the important aerobic weight lifting part of the workout. During this 15-minute aerobic warm-up you should target 80% of your predicted maximum heart rate for age as your target level. (Maximum Heart Rate (MHR) using Miller Formula: MHR = 217- (0.85 x age).) Once you finish the 15-minute warm-up, the real workout begins. You now have one minute to get to the first set of weight lifting. You will be working pretty hard and non-stop for the next 20-25 minutes.

AEROBIC CIRCUIT TRAINING

Once you finish your warm-up you will begin the weight lifting part of the workout. The key point of this weight-training workout is that it can be done by anyone! You do not have to be a gymnast, ballet dancer or world-class athlete to do this. All of the exercises outlined in this book can be done by "average," and

34

overweight adults. These same exercises (with more weight and/or more reps) will still be highly effective once you are trained, super-fit, and thinner.

One of the critical points about this weight training session is to do this aerobically. This means that you should be breathing hard, and have an elevated heart rate throughout the weight lifting the workout. This aerobic component of the weight lifting will increase stress to the muscles during the session. In this way, you can get a more profound training effect in the muscles while lifting less weight and doing fewer sets of repetitive weight lifting, and in less time. This approach also lets you build your aerobic fitness simultaneously with your weight training. This is a highly efficient workout. "Two for the price of one."

In order to do this aerobically it is important that you minimize the rest between the weight lifting sets. If you are just starting out and have never worked out, you may need as much as one minute of rest between the weight lifting sets. The other "trick" as you are just starting out will be making sure that you are lifting the right amount of weight for each set. We will address the question of, *What is the right amount of weight?* in a section to follow shortly. Eventually the rest between sets should only be about 10-20 seconds, and just long enough to move from one set of dumbbells or piece of exercise equipment to the next in the current circuit. This is aerobic.

I want to make a few quick comments about breathing. Do not hold your breath while you are weight lifting. Yes, you need to breathe during this workout. Work on rhythmic and strong breathing. When you are lifting the weight or contracting the muscle group(s) make certain to time this with strong exhalation. This will enhance you strength and make the workout a little easier. Be conscious of, and focus on your breathing throughout the workout.

I want to distinguish the Burn Calories approach from the more usual civilized type of weight lifting that I typically see when I observe individuals, with or without their personal trainers, at the gym. That workout goes something like this: "OK Susan, let's start with 15 repetitions of this biceps exercise." "Great job!" "Hey Susan how is your friend Joan? I haven't seen her at the gym lately..., did you see that latest Ben Affleck movie that came out last week? Yada, yada, yada." "OK. Are you rested? Great. Let's go over and do some squats, etc. etc." There is no time for gossip and book reviews during the Burn Calories workout. It may not be P90X (hard core and extreme "fad" workout for super-fit adults), but the principles of keeping it aerobic and continuous is very important to the muscle stressing and training effect that we are seeking.

Although there are some great personal trainers, with many trainers they do not want to push their clients too hard, or make it at all painful. They are worried that if they make it painful the client will not come back for another training session. In addition, many clients will not confess to their trainer that the weight was too light and it did not really "burn." They just want to look good in front of their trainer. There is some discomfort required if you are going to adequately stress the skeletal muscle to turn on the cell signals to remodel the muscle, build new mitochondria, etc. So, in some ways it is better to choose the weights and number of reps yourself. Only you know if there is some "pain" in the muscle fibers at the end of the set. As you have head a million times, "no pain, no gain." Here is the good news. The workout is quite short and the benefits of this brief stress and pain to the muscle will pay huge metabolic dividends.

The aerobic weight lifting of every major muscle group is best done in circuits. A circuit will consist of exercises to focus on two or three key muscle groups at a time. In circuit training we move from an exercise focused on one muscle group, and then immediately to another exercise focusing on a second muscle group, etc.

There are two main reasons that we focus on a "circuit" training approach. The first is that it is a little less boring. More importantly, we want to give the first stressed muscle group a couple of minutes to recover. However, we do not want you to rest for a couple of minutes waiting for that muscle group to recover in order to do another set. This workout is non-stop. In order to keep it aerobic, with virtually no rest between weight lifting sets, and to give each muscle group a little recovery we have to move to another muscle group in a circuit, before going back to re-stress the first muscle group.

What does this mean? The best way to explain this is to give an example. In Table 3 we have defined the ten key muscle groups to be exercised in every Burn Calories workout. There are other muscles that will get recruited and trained alongside these key muscle groups. We are focusing on these ten muscle groups to keep it a little simpler. Each circuit will consist of 10-30 repetitions of exercises, for two or three of these muscle groups, done sequentially. For example, you could start with a focus on biceps and triceps. You will do 10-15 reps of a biceps exercise. You get 15-30 seconds of rest, followed by 10-15 reps of a triceps exercise. You get another 15-30 seconds of rest followed by 10-15 reps of the biceps exercise, and then finishing this "circuit" with 15 more reps of the triceps. You can now cross these two muscle groups off the list. You have eight more muscle groups to go.

38

You may ask, "How many reps (repetitions) should I do for each exercise?" This is a good question. The answer is it will depend on your level of skeletal muscle strength and the weight you are lifting, or exercise that you are doing. This is the only critical thing: It must hurt and burn in your muscle(s) during the last 3-4 reps. This burning or pain in the muscle is the sign of severe muscle stress that *will* lead to the adaptation that we are looking for in the skeletal muscle. If it is too easy and it does not hurt, there will be little change in your skeletal muscle cells, and you will be just burning calories while you sweat, but not altering, and restructuring muscle fibers in order to "Burn Calories While You Sleep." So remember, if you make it burn it (the skeletal muscle) will learn. It will remodel, build fibers, become stronger and burn more basal metabolic calories.

Let's get back to the actual workout. These circuits are may be most efficient if they contain antagonistic muscle groups, such as biceps and triceps, or quadriceps and hamstrings. The circuits may include a third muscle group. You should not have more than three focused (main) muscle groups in any one circuit, because this will give too much rest to each stressed muscle group. You can appreciate that the maximum number of these circuits is five circuits (2 muscle groups per circuit = the 10 muscle groups on the list). If you keep your rest on pace, and do two sets with each exercise that day for a particular muscle group, this entire weight

39

lifting workout will go quickly (20-30 minutes). You could accelerate the training effect, at the expense of lengthening the workout by approximately 10 minutes, if you do three sets with each muscle group, instead of two sets.

In general, you can choose any order or combination of key muscle groups to create these circuits, and any one of several exercises to focus on a given muscle group (e.g., triceps will be stressed with "tricep pull downs" or "dips" or "kickbacks" with dumbbells (page 59). Certain exercises will stress more than one key muscle group at a time, even though that exercise may be "focused" on a particular muscle group. (e.g., dead lift for hamstrings, shown on page 57, will stress mainly hamstrings, but will also stress gluteus, biceps, chest and upper and lower back). This multi-muscle approach is intended to increase the aerobic intensity, and to increase the high intensity and repeated muscle stress to each major muscle group, in order to maximize the stress, that will promote muscle remodeling. Fair warning, though. These multi-muscle key exercises are more tiring, stressful and aerobic. It is a key concept of this workout, no matter how you choose to "personalize" it, to maximize skeletal muscle stress, create repeated high intensity stress on every major muscle group, and promote aerobic fitness, simultaneously.

For those readers who have never worked out with weights before, there are photo sequences demonstrating many of the key types of exercise to stress different muscle groups. The exercises shown are not meant to show an exhaustive list of all exercises for any given muscle group. Further information, alternative exercises can be found in numerous exercise books, or better yet, working with a talented personal trainer. There is at least one option for each muscle group exercise that can be done with minimal equipment, and at home using the list of equipment shown in Table 3. You do not have to buy an expensive membership at a fancy health club to do this. Many of these exercises require little or no exercise equipment other than free weights (dumbbells), or a floor, a mat or a chair or bench and a wall.

In addition to the exercises for every muscle group there are three key Burn Calories workout exercises that, ideally, you should incorporate into every workout (shown with an * in the photo sequences). Ideally, these should be included in every Burn Calories workout. These are amazing multi-muscle exercises that are aerobic, and are focused on key large muscle groups such as chest and shoulders, butt (gluteus) and hamstrings, and inner and outer thighs and lateral abdominal muscles. We will call these three exercises *The Key Three.* Learn these three exercises and incorporate 15-20 reps of each of the three in every workout and it will pay huge dividends. (see * in photo sequences).

41

In the photo sequences and the associated figure legends below, I have outlined depicted what I call the "Classic" Burn Calories workout. This describes the exact sequence and sets that I have developed for my personal workout routine to create high intensity and repetitive stress on virtually every major muscle group. It includes a lot of crunches, as you might expect from an abdominal strength freak like me. This is a very efficient, but (fair warning) challenging workout. Although many trainers like to mix it up, with 4-5 different exercise routines for each muscle group in different workouts, I personally like having a set routine, that hits every muscle group (and many muscle groups 2-3 times during the workout), uses all of the key multi-muscle exercises, achieves a very high level of aerobic stress, and gets me out of the gym 20-25 minutes after my warm-up. This is super-efficient, and I encourage all of the readers to try this "Classic" routine at least once. If you like it, as I do, then you will have a reproducible routine with a very fixed time commitment. If you like to mix it up that is also fine as long as you follow the basic guidelines for the Burn Calories workout that is best summarized in the Table at the end of this chapter. Ultimately you may create your own, and personalized "Classic" routine, that incorporates all of the basic principles of the Burn Calories workout.

Every Muscle Group Every Workout

As outlined above, every workout will contain at least two sets of exercises to stress every major muscle group. Unlike some exercise plans that suggest that you focus on one muscle group or region (like lower body or legs, or arms) in a given workout, it is very important for this program that every workout is a whole body workout. Every major muscle group will be stressed in every workout! If we stress every major muscle group every second or third day your whole body fitness will proceed on an even pace. All of your muscle groups and individual muscles will get stronger, rebuild muscle fibers in better synchrony, and this will create a larger and more rapid cumulative impact on the changes in your metabolism.

As described above, it probably makes relatively little difference which muscle groups come first versus last, although there will be more stress on the muscle groups that are trained at the end of the workout, when energy stores are more depleted. At the end of the workout the stresses on the muscles are more profound and bordering on anaerobic. Since the larger muscle groups, like the back and abdominals are more important to the net change in your core metabolism and your core strength, I recommend that the workout ends with major stress to these larger muscle groups. This may make the workout a little harder, but will pay earlier dividends with regard to the acceleration of changes in your metabolic rate.

What is the "Right" Amount of Weight?

This is a very important question. The right amount of weight to use for each exercise is critical for everyone who does this workout, from beginners, all the way to very fit individuals that have strength and prior experience with weight lifting. The right amount of weight is the weight that makes the last 3-4 repetitions in each 10-20 repetition set hurt and burn a bit. If you are using so little weight that it is really easy, with no discomfort at the end of the set, and/or you are not breathing pretty hard after the set, then you need to use more weight, or do more reps. Conversely, if you cannot complete at least 10 repetitions of the exercise you should back off on the weight. As you start out you can quickly determine what the correct starting weight is for you. Everyone will have their own starting set point for the amount of weight it takes for a given exercise to be aerobic, stressful and hurting during the last 3-4 reps.

The other critical point is that over time, you should expect to get stronger, which will require you to increase the amount of weight that is required to stress each muscle group. For example, a beginner woman might be stressed to do 15 reps with 5 pounds with a biceps curl when she first starts this workout program. If she sticks with the workout 2-3 days per week, we would expect her to need 8-10 pounds to get the same "burn" on the 15th rep after 3-4 months. She will eventually plateau, depending on age, genetics, etc. at perhaps 12-15 pounds. After one year of doing this program regularly the correct amount of weight for each individual will begin to stabilize. That is, you are doing this workout three times per week, and you still get fatigue in your muscles at the same weight that you were using 2 months ago. Since this is not body building, at this point you can stop increasing the weights. You may slowly increase the number of reps as you get more fit over time. For some exercises, like calf raises, it may take 30-50 reps to get a "burn." So, just remember the key is to make the last 3-5 reps "burn" or hurt a bit. That is the signal that you are achieving the high intensity muscle stress that is required to trigger the muscle remodeling and metabolic changes we are targeting.

Each individual will eventually reach equilibrium at certain weights for each exercise. At this point you should have increased your strength and lean muscle mass by 20-40%. When combined with the reasonable eating habits described in Chapter Five, you will begin to reach your target weight. We will talk more about this later.

FOCUS ON THE BIG MUSCLES; ESPECIALLY ABDOMINALS

Where are most of the calories burned? They are burned in the big muscles! Although the Burn Calories workout is intended to work virtually every muscle group in every workout, the workout is intended to place extra focus of muscle stress upon the largest muscle groups (see Table). We want symmetry to your new and fit body, which is why we want to work all of your muscles.

However, the main metabolic changes occur by the constant stressing and remodeling of the largest muscles. This makes sense. No matter how much stress we place on the muscles in your index finger or even the smaller muscles of your forearm, this will have little impact on your whole body basal metabolic rate. This is analogous to fuel burning in automobiles. If you are driving a huge Chevy Tahoe or other large SUV (your large abdominal core muscles) you will be burning a lot of gasoline, even when the engine is in idol. Conversely, if you are driving a small hybrid like a Toyota Prius, (like triceps or calf muscles) you will be burning relatively little gasoline while driving or in idol. If we want to burn a lot of calories while we sleep we need the recruitment of a lot of muscle mass. These large muscles also burn a lot more calories during the workout (burning calories while you sweat), which is also a good thing. This is why we will focus so much on these large muscles, especially the abdominal muscles, during the workout and in other ways on our off days.

MORE ABOUT ABDOMINAL MUSCLE (CRUNCHES IN YOUR CAR)

The most important of the large muscle groups are the abdominal muscles. The abdominal muscles consist of pairs (right and left side) of muscles. The main abdominal muscles are the rectus abdominus (muscles in the front that give that "six-pack"), the transversus abdominus, and internal and external oblique muscles on the sides. When they are stressed, these are some of the most metabolically active muscles in your body. I view these muscles as the key glucose burning system in the body. When you get these muscles in action one should visualize, and will actually sense, the fuel burning that is going on in this energy/glucose-burning factory.

Equally important is the critical role that these muscles play in what has commonly been referred to as core strength. These muscles are critical to your entire body strength, balance and overall fitness. Super strong abdominal muscles will make you more athletic, let you lift things without herniating a disc in your lower back, and make you more athletic in every way. It will also make you look much better, both with and without clothes on. This is why the program outlined in this book is so focused on stressing and rebuilding incredibly fit strong abdominal muscles.

In the Burn Calories workout we have stressed the importance of working the upper, lower and side abdominal muscles. Every Burn Calories workout should include major abdominal work as outlined in the workout and in the pictorial section. However, the real key to creating and maintaining extraordinary abdominal muscles, and the associated alteration of metabolic rate and core strength is the abdominal work that is done every day outside of the regular workout.

Don't faint now. I want you to do at least 2,000 crunches per week every week for the rest of your life! You are thinking, *This guy is insane. That would take me five hours a week!* Once you calm down, I am going to tell you just how easy this is. It will take virtually no additional time out of your day.

What am I talking about? I am talking about doing crunches in bed before you get up every morning (40-75 crunches), 80-150 crunches in your car going to work (40-75 crunches x 2 sets), and 80-150 coming home from work (40-75 x 2 sets), crunches or leg lifts (lower abdominal muscle work 20-40) every night before you go to sleep. OK, let's add those up. That is 50 crunches before you get out of bed, 100 driving to work (or driving on errands during weekend) and 100 driving home, and 30-

50 before you go to bed. That is 280 crunches/day or 1,960 crunches per week. Let's add to that the 200-300 abdominal crunches and leg lifts in each 40-minute Burn Calories workout, three times per week (i.e., another 600-900 crunches per week). Now we are at 2,560-3,000 crunches per week! If you are really motivated, and as your abdominal muscles get much stronger, you can do another 1,000-2,000 a week (4-5,000 total/week) with virtually no much additional time or effort taken out of your day. When you do this, the program will pay dividends even faster.

It is almost embarrassing how little real time it takes to add this activity (crunches in your car, etc.) to your daily routine. I am talking about taking as little as 3-5 minutes a day do these 300-500 crunches/day during time when you are really doing very little productively (i.e., you are just driving to work or sitting at your desk). This is one of the key magic tricks to the sustainable change in metabolism, fitness and weight loss taught in this book. Let's use this otherwise *wasted time* to build core strength and permanently transform your metabolic rate. This rather trivial alteration in your otherwise boring morning drive to work will additively enhance metabolic rate, build core strength, and may even prevent a herniated disc that would have happened next year!

And, of course you can do these sitting crunches at home or at work at your desk, on an airplane, or anywhere or anytime that you are bored and thinking how much thinner, and fitter you want to be. You can imagine based on these numbers as outlined, that it would actually be pretty easy to do 3,000 or even 4,000 crunches per week, if you spent less than 1% of your time wasted in the car, at the airport, in the library, at your desk, etc. The more you do the faster and more dramatic will be the result.

I do need to give you one warning about these crunches. Be careful to not make it too obvious or grimace too much, especially while you are stuck at a red light, so the person in the car next to you does not think you are either having some major gastrointestinal problem or a sexual encounter while driving. Probably best not to do this while sitting next to a police car as well.

Lastly, you are probably asking, "What on earth does he mean? How do you do abdominal crunches in your car while driving?" It is very easy. The "sitting crunch," as I call it is shown workout photos (page 61). The key elements to doing this effectively are, 1) place one hand (not both hands because you are driving, stupid), gently on your abdominal muscles; 2) over a 1-3 second interval contract all of your abdominal muscles as hard as you possibly can while moving your chest and shoulders slightly forward (feel them contract like steel with your hand to maximize the contraction), and then 3) relax the muscles completely. Then repeat this. There should be only a 1-2 second rest between crunches. When you do this properly you will really feel it. It will burn! If you are not feeling it you are not contracting the muscles hard enough. We are talking intense contraction. Imagine someone is about to punch you in the stomach as hard as they can, and you need to protect yourself by massively contracting every abdominal muscle fiber. That is how hard each contraction should be. At first, you may only be able to do 20-30 of these in a row without feeling the pain of the lactic acid buildup in your untrained abdominal muscles. After 6-9 months, you will be able to easily do strong sets of 40-50 sitting crunches at a time. After 2 years I now routinely have to do 100-110 per set to get to fatigue and burning pain. When you jump up from sets of 30 to sets of 80 crunches in your car, that is when you will know your strength and metabolic rate is transforming.

For women (see Chapter Ten) who are worried about getting a six-pack that may not be "feminine," let's cross that bridge when we get there. When your husband or significant other says, "Hey Babe, you are really getting too buffed! That six-pack of yours is a bit intimidating," only then you can worry about cutting back on your abdominal work. When that happens please send me an email or a letter—or even better, a picture! So, until someone complains that you look too "buffed" and muscular, you need to try to trust me and stick with this program. It will work. No excuses from the girls. You can benefit just as much—if not more—as the boys from crunches in your car.

Other "Off Day" Pearls: Isometric Fidgeting and Other Ways to Burn Calories

This tip is about burning more calories while you are awake, but also continuing the high intensity muscle contractions that will stimulate muscle growth and the ongoing metabolic transformation of your muscle. The key concept in this part of the program is to use otherwise wasted, sedentary time throughout your day to enhance muscle strength, accelerate the muscle remodeling that is being triggered by the core Burn Calories workout, enhance training of your muscles and accelerate weight loss.

I have made up the name "isometric fidgeting" for the novel approach that I have developed to accelerate your training and calorie burning. First let's touch on fidgeting. Fidgeting is defined as the act of moving about restlessly. We all know people who do this. You may have noticed that most fidgeters are thin. Indeed, studies have shown that people who fidget are, on the average, much thinner than their non-fidgeting counterparts. I find people who fidget a little annoying. That is why I have invented the concept of isometric fidgeting.

Isometric means without movement. In isometric fidgeting you strongly contract one or muscle group repetitively, but without much, if any movement or motion of the muscle. So we are talking about strongly contracting a muscle or muscle group repetitively, but without motion, during the day (e.g., triceps). Since you are not jumping about, you can do this pretty unobtrusively. This activity is the equivalent of the crunches in your car (meant for your abdominal muscles) but in this case to stress "other" muscle groups. The best muscle groups to focus on for isometric contractions (fidgeting) are your gluteus (butt) muscles, triceps, biceps and quadriceps. One could also do this with calf muscles, back muscles (like latissimus dorsi), etc.

How often should you do this? I would recommend doing 5-15 strong isometric contractions of each of the above muscle groups at least once or twice per day. The more that you do this, the faster you will train these muscle groups. These isometric stresses are even more stressful when you do this on the same day as one of your Burn Calories workouts, since this gives even more stress to these muscle groups. If you do 1-2 sets of 15 contractions of each of these 4 muscle groups every day, this should only take about 5-6 minutes per day. Just like crunches in your car, this can be done during times when you are probably not doing anything productive anyway. This contributes to the incredible time-efficiency of this approach to getting thin and transforming your metabolism.

EXERCISE EQUIPMENT NEEDED FOR DOING THIS AT HOME

Ideally, one will start this program using a health club facility. These health clubs range from modest and affordable to very fancy and very expensive. See if there is a club that meets you needs in your area. The good thing about joining the health club is that they generally will have all of the equipment and space that you need to do this workout efficiently. You will also have access to personal trainers who can be very helpful especially if you have never done weight lifting, to make sure that you form is correct. Weight lifting done with completely wrong technique will net much less benefit and training effect. Form and pace of the lifting is critical. If you just throw the weights up and let gravity drop the weight you will not be stressing the muscle through the entire range of motion and this may reduce the training effect of that exercise by 50%. Slow and controlled in perfect form is key. This is best learned by either working with a personal trainer for 2-5 sessions.

The alternative to joining a health club is to make your own workout space in your home or apartment. Even without access to a health club, there are at least 2-3 exercises for each muscle group, and the 3 key exercises (*) that can be done in each Burn Calories workout in your home. The exercises for each key muscle group that can easily be done in a modest home gym, with very little investment of space or dollars.

Table 3 lists all of the equipment needed to do this workout at home. It basically consists of a set of free weights (dumbbells) that are suited in range of weights for your initial level of strength and training. This will also be different, in general, for men than for women. Men will probably need to start with a higher weight range of dumbbells than women. Other than these weights, you need a flat area to place a workout mat or towel, and some form of a rigid bench. The best bench would be the kind that you might buy at a local sporting goods store for about $50. If you have the money and interest, you can purchase a piece of cardio equipment. I personally recommend an elliptical machine that incorporates arm exercise. A treadmill, stationary bicycle, stair climber or treadmill can also be used. There are dozens of fancy "abdominal" machines marketed in infomercials or findable on the web. Some of these are pretty good and may help beginners do their crunches with better form and less neck strain. Most of these are fine, but plain old crunches, done with proper form, especially on a reverse incline bench, is about as good as it gets.

Routine

... "CLASSIC" BURN CALORIES WORKOUT

The workout goes as follows:

1) 12-15 minutes aerobic warm-up, ideally on machine that gets most muscle groups and low impact. I like elliptical trainer that incorporates arms.

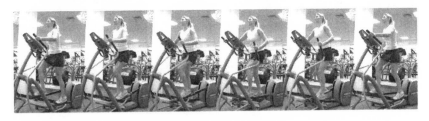

ELIPTICAL TRAINER

2) Immediately move to weight lifting, in circuits, with no more than 15-30 seconds between sets, and two sets of each of the exercises as listed below. Except as noted you usually do 15-20 reps for each set. The amount of weight is chosen so that the last 3-4 reps are very challenging and burn. If the last reps do not hurt, it is too little weight. Every individual will be different with regard to the amount of weight that will make these 15 reps high intensity.

3) First circuit has 4 exercises: Start with bicep curls with as much weight as you can (as above) for 15 reps.

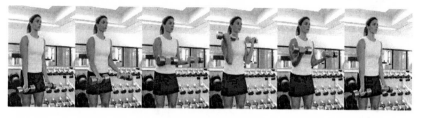

BICEP CURL

4) Using same weights held in hands, standing up, keep legs straight and bend from waist to touch the weights to the floor and then lift straight up lifting weights with arms straight to standing position, (Dead Man Lift); this gets hamstrings, lower back, calf and gluteus muscle groups), pulling chest back as you stand tall with weights held at your side (pectoral and deltoid and trapezius) muscles. You repeat this 15 times.

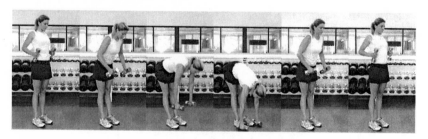

DEAD MAN LIFT*

5) Immediately after this you hold weights straight down at your side and bending laterally letting weight in one arm drop along outside of your leg as far as you can (weight/hand may get to about level of knee), then with arms still straight bending laterally the other way with the weight in the other hand along the opposite leg.

This gets mainly lateral abdominal muscles, and a little bit in biceps and deltoids and adductors and abductors of inner and outer thighs. This is 20-25 reps counting left + right as one rep.

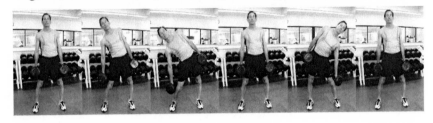

Lateral Abs *

6) Exercise #4 in this set is triceps, best done as a pull down with one of the machines with weight stacks, since this also gets trapezius (back) and some shoulders. Alternatives are "Kick Backs" or "Dips." After this, repeat 3-6 for the second set in this circuit.

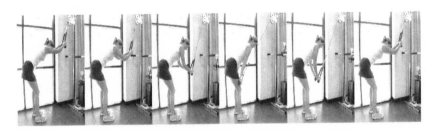

Tricep Pull Down

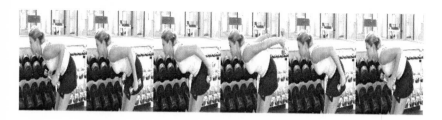

KICK BACKS

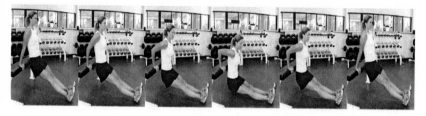

DIPS

7) The next circuit is calf, chest and abdominals. Start with calf raises (Photoset 6). Standing on one foot, you can gently hold onto something and then do 50-70 calf raises on one leg, followed immediately by the other leg.

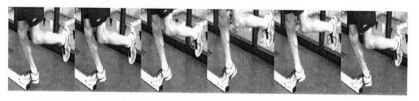

CALF RAISE

8) Next move immediately to do chest presses either with machine or free weights (Dumbell Chest press in other pictures set) of barbell for 15 reps on chest (remember last 3-4 reps are hard then very hard).

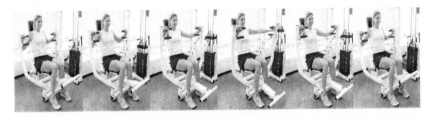

CHEST PRESS

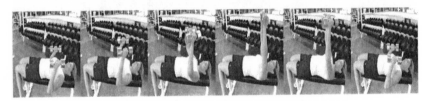

CHEST PRESS WITH DUMBELLS

9) Immediately after the chest presses, do crunches in sitting or lying position. You will do as many as you can until the last 4-5 really burn, contracting every abdominal muscle fiber as hard as you can with each crunch. Sitting position is same as the crunches in your car as described in the book. (Remember that you need to do 200-300 crunches every day on your off-days, in sets of 50-70 at a time).

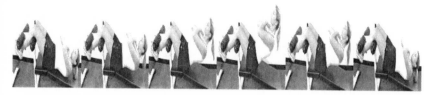

CRUNCH IN LYING POSITION

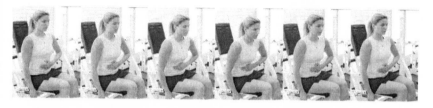

SITTING CRUNCH ("CRUNCHES IN YOUR CAR")

10) After doing these 50-70 crunches, you immediately do another set of 15 chest presses. Following this you do another set of 50-70 crunches. Then immediately back to do your second set of calf raises. That ends this circuit.

11) The next circuit is quadriceps and abdominals. You move to either leg extension machine or leg press machine to focus on quadriceps. You do 15 reps using the 13, 14 15 rule (i.e., it really hurts for last three reps). Then another set of 50-70 sitting crunches (while sitting). Then 30 seconds rest and another set of leg extensions or leg press; then another set of crunches. That ends this circuit.

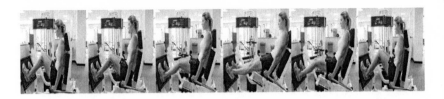

LEG PRESS

12) The last circuit begins with free weight in each hand. Generally this will use 5-20 pounds of weight for you. You start with weights held with straight arms in front of you and low, then with arms straight lift both arms straight up and together in front of your face and straight up in the air, then still with straight arms, all the way away from your body to the side and down to lower weights to your side, then low and in front of you, then straight up again, (this is one circular rep). You repeat this (gets chest, deltoids, biceps, triceps) 15 times. This is a great exercise.

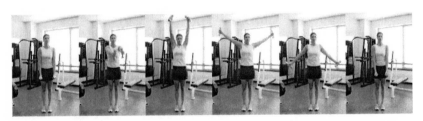

CHEST CIRCLES *

13) Immediately following the "Chest Circles" (15 seconds rest), begin lateral raises for 12-15 reps.

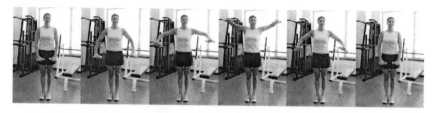

LATERAL RAISE

14) Then, immediately move to lower back extension using the lower back (stationary machine) or the lower back machine that moves with weights. Do 15-25 reps of lower back extension. This back extension machine also gets your hamstrings and your gluteus muscles.

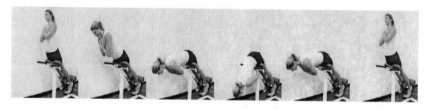

LOWER BACK EXTENSION

15) Immediately go to tilted inclined bench made for sit-ups. With head down and feet wrapped at top of incline bench you will do as many crunches as you can, with the first half with alternating lateral crunches and the last half as straight incline bench crunches.

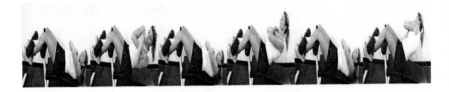

LATERAL CRUNCH

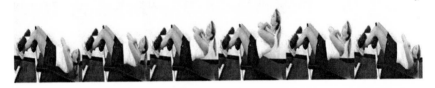

STRAIGHT CRUNCH

16) Repeat 12-14 for the second set. Then do straight leg lifts using the same incline bench (15-20 would be good here). This is the last exercise. You are done. This is very aerobic if done properly.

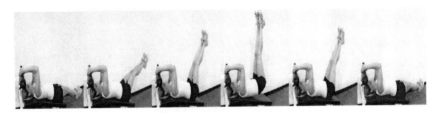

STRAIGHT LEG LIFT

This entire workout, including a 12 minute warm-up, takes about 35-40 minutes. It may take you 45-50 minutes if you take a little more rest as you get started. I am hopeful that you will appreciate the high intensity training (HIT), and aerobic nature of this, but also the short duration and time efficiencies of this type of workout. Other variations are, of course (see other Photosets for alternative or substitute exercise for different muscle groups), possible using the primary goal to get high intensity muscle stress (HIT) and hit every muscle group. As per the book it is also important to do high intensity muscle contraction of muscle groups (like triceps, quadriceps, gluteus) on your off days (isometric fidgeting), and the extra 300-400 crunches (in your car) every day. This will amplify the HIT effect in the skeletal muscles, especially when done on your workout days (3 days/week).

It is important to acknowledge that this exact set of exercises is not the only way to achieve the goals of a "Burn Calories" workout. There are many other combinations and exercise options that can create the correct full body, metabolism altering stress on all of your key muscle groups. Be creative. Do what works for you Work with a personal trainer for your first 3-4 workouts if you can afford it. As long as it is virtually non-stop (15-30 seconds between sets) and aerobic, creates HIT and muscle stress for all muscle groups, has at least two sets of every muscle group exercise and incorporates at least 200-300 crunches in the workout, you will achieve the goals, and change your metabolic rate. You will begin to "Burn Calories While You Sleep."

TABLE 3

EQUIPMENT TO DO "BURN CALORIES" WORKOUT AT HOME

1) Ideally, a piece of aerobic exercise equipment (i.e., elliptical, stationary bicycle, treadmill, rowing machine, etc.) (Not required).

2) A floor.

3) A wall.

4) An exercise bench, flat, or with adjustable slant, or a hard chair.

5) Free weights (dumbbells) ranging from 5 lbs. to as much as 30-60 lbs. depending on your level of strength and fitness.

6) Water and a towel, and ideally a music source.

TABLE 4

KEY MUSCLE GROUPS (IN ORDER OF IMPORTANCE)

1) Abdominals (rectus abdominus, tranversus and obliques)

2) Upper back (trapezius and others)

3) Chest (pectoral and others)

4) Lower back and gluteus (butt)

5) Quadriceps

6) Shoulders (deltoids and others)

7) Hamstrings

8) Biceps

9) Calves

10) Triceps

CHAPTER THREE

KEY RULES FOR "THE BURN CALORIES" WORKOUT

1) 40-45 minutes 2-3 times per week. This is religion!

2) Being "busy" or traveling is not an excuse for breaking Rule 1!

3) Warm up aerobically (10-15 minutes).

4) Aerobic circuit training for your weight lifting (20-25 minutes).

5) 15-20 reps, every muscle group, every workout, last three reps hurt!

6) There is NO rest (30 seconds between sets). It is aerobic!

7) Focus on the BIG muscles!

8) Abs, abs and more abs (at least 2,000 crunches per week (in your car!)

9) Isometric exercises whenever you can. Isometric fidgeting!

10) Be active (walk the stairs, play tennis, ski, skate, hike, swim).

❧ *Chapter Four* ❧

Aerobic Fitness: Still Important But Let's Stop the Two Hours on a Treadmill Routine!

I am not a gym rat. I try not to spend more time than needed in the gym. That is how I discovered the efficiency of the Burn Calories aerobic weight lifting approach. However, I have spent enough time at the fitness club to make one interesting observation. The people with the most weight to lose (i.e., heaviest men and women) are more often than not working out on the treadmill, or the elliptical or stationary bicycle, etc. If you go and talk to these folks and ask them about their working out on the treadmill, they will generally tell you that they do it 3-4 times per week, for at least 45-60 minutes per workout. If you ask them why they are doing it, they will generally say, to lose weight. If you then ask them what their weight was six months ago compared to today, they will usually say about the same. Somehow, they have not figured it out. The key take home message in this chapter is that unless you have 12-15 hours a week to spend on workout machines, long, slow workouts on the treadmill, elliptical, etc. will not solve your weight problem. This type of workout, in general, only *"burns calories while you sweat"* and not while you sleep. It will not stress your skeletal muscles enough to alter your metabolic rate.

Many people believe that the key to getting thin is to spend more hours walking on the treadmill. They reason that this will burn off the weight that they gained over Thanksgiving, Christmas, etc. Some folks even get motivated to start this for the first time after a food binging holiday. They are sixty pounds overweight, and just added six more pounds over Christmas. They join a health club. They step on the treadmill and begin to repent for their eating sins. They start up this modern wonder of calibrated, electronically monitored workouts. They start walking and, with some effort, maintain a 2.5 miles per hour walking pace. They do this for forty-five minutes. Now they are exhausted, and sweaty. Surely this is the path to salvation. They look at the calorie counter on the state-of-the-art treadmill machine. It reads "317 calories." They feel good about themselves and go home to tell their spouse about their incredible new religion of fitness.

When they get home they are hungry and crack open that new box of Toll House cookies. Just out of curiosity, they check the side of the box, only to discover that one large chocolate chip cookie has 210 calories! This really pisses them off. They realize that they just spent close to an hour sweating on a treadmill, and all they got was enough burning calories while they sweated to burn

High intensity short duration

off one and a half cookies. That is when they decide to get a refund from the health club and forget about those silly treadmills. They give up completely and proceed to eat the whole box of cookies to reward themselves for realizing that exercise is just a waste of time. Does this sound familiar?

Don't get me wrong. I really believe that working out aerobically is important. There is no question that pounding on the treadmill, or elliptical, or jogging, swimming have major benefits compared to doing nothing. The main problem with these types of exercise is that they do not efficiently or adequately stress your skeletal muscles. Most of these forms of exercise also do not stress every muscle group. This type of exercise will not really train and stress your large and critical core muscles, such as the abdominal muscles.

These activities will improve your stamina, and will burn calories, but will have much less impact upon your basal metabolic rate than aerobic (high intensity-short duration) weight lifting. With a treadmill, you are only modestly stressing your calf, and leg muscles, and not much else. As I have said, when you walking on a treadmill, pedaling on a stationary bike, walking, or even jogging, is basically only burning calories while you sweat. In contrast, during a Burn Calories workout you will burn more calories in a shorter time during the workout once you get to your plateau weights (about 600-800 calories in 40 minutes). This is also a great aerobic and <u>whole body</u> workout. You will get stamina and fitness from the aerobic warm up and the (aerobic) weight lifting. Importantly you are stressing your large core muscles. It is estimated that you will burn another 500-1,000 calories in the next forty-eight hours after the Burn Calories workout as your skeletal muscles recover, and remodel the muscle fibers in response to the stress of the aerobic weight lifting. So after a high intensity, muscle stressing workout, like that described in the Burn Calories workout, you will receive huge dividends or interest on the workout investment, particularly compared to the boring, walk on treadmill exercise.

So do you want to invest your precious time in the treadmill/exercise bike/walking investment, that pays little or no interest (i.e., does not burn calories for the next 24-48 hours after the workout) or invest in a workout that will continue to pay calorie burning dividends after you have completed the workout? Do you want to change your basic metabolic rate and Burn Calories While You Sleep, or walk on a treadmill and only burn calories while you sweat? The answer should be obvious. The program outlined in Chapter Three is amazingly time efficient. The whole workout takes 40% less time than the fellow just spent 60 minutes on the treadmill getting his religion. Do you want to put your money in the bank and get 2% dividends (treadmills/ burn calories while you sweat), or get 70-80% dividends by transforming and growing your skeletal muscle (burning calories while you sleep)? If the above scenario resonates with you, it is time for you to change your religion, stop sweating for two hours on the treadmill, and get ready to get thin and fit.

One final word on the subject, in case you treadmill lovers are angry with me. I am not saying that slow treadmill or other fitness activities are a terrible thing to do. If you love to spend an hour and a half on the treadmill every day, that is fine. Some people find it relaxing and enjoyable. It is burning calories, and it sure beats the hell out of sitting on the couch, drinking beer, and eating potato chips while you watch a Seinfeld rerun. It just is *not* the key to efficient success in losing weight.

Similarly, enhancing your aerobic fitness with other fun activities will pay dividends. Playing tennis, racket ball, soccer, basketball, volleyball, swimming, jogging (with some limits to protect your joints), climbing, hiking, biking, dancing, martial arts, yoga, skiing, Pilates, etc. are all great and fun ways to enhance your fitness, your aerobic health. These activities are encouraged, and they will burn calories and help you to achieve your weight loss goals. The key messaging is that these are great, fun, and calorie burning. They are not a substitute for the high-intensity muscle stress achieved as the core of the Burn Calories program, which is designed to more profoundly rev up your resting metabolic rate, build new muscle fibers and enhance core strength.

Chapter Four Key Points: Aerobic Fitness

1) Aerobic fitness is important and will improve stamina and overall fitness.

2) Spending many hours/week on cardio equipment is time consuming, AND

3) 4-5 hours/week treadmill will not lead to sustained weight loss.

4) Slow paced cardio equipment workouts do not create "fit" muscle.

5) Slow paced cardio equipment workouts do not impact metabolic rate.

6) Spending time on "cardio" equipment only burns calories while you sweat.

7) Aerobic fitness is best achieved with intense, aerobic weight lifting.

8) This aerobic fitness can be further improved with "fun" athletic activities such as basketball, tennis, racket ball, dancing, martial arts, etc.

❧ *Chapter Five* ❧

LIFETIME DIETARY HABITS: WHY AMERICA IS FAT BUT YOU DON'T HAVE TO BE!

L ook around us. Mega meals, value packs, two-for-one meals, huge portions, triple-whoppers, fried foods, stir-in fresh ice-cream stores, etc. Food is everywhere and in quantities and portions that are meant for an everyday feast. We finish a huge meal and they offer us the dessert menu with eight unbelievable and super-sized desserts. We are programmed genetically to eat at all times when there are feasting conditions, so we eat even when we are not hungry and long after we are full. We love those fried foods, fatty foods and especially those sweet carbohydrate treats like cookies, cake, and candy. The land of plenty has made us a land of obesity. How can we reverse this epidemic of over-eating?

The last chapter outlined a powerful tool to increase our everyday metabolism so that we can eat a reasonable amount of food and still lose weight. If we can increase your basal metabolic rate by 40-50% and modulate eating, this will lead to success. In fact, this is the most important chapter in the book! If you follow and adopt the eating "rules" in this chapter, it will have a huge impact.

A lot of books have, in my opinion, have gone too far in prescribing complicated regimens, dietary lists, hundreds of specific weight loss recipes, and rigid calorie counting or other schemes. Fad diets often take it a step further, to regimens that are scientifically unproven, expensive and rarely sustainable.

In this book, we are taking a more common sense approach to control of eating. The goal is to make your conscious and logical mind dictate your daily eating habits, rather than boredom or your emotional mind. Critics will say this is too simple and simple minded, and that it will never work. "People already know the rules of eating that you are proposing." There is some truth to this. I believe that every one of the rules of eating outlined in this chapter have been mentioned in some place in almost every fitness and weight loss book before. However, I do not believe that they have been organized into a simple mantra in a way that, hopefully, can be imbedded or ingrained in your conscious and unconscious mind as your day-to-day rules for eating. The intention here is to get that little voice in the back of your head to say, "I am not hungry. I won't eat," or "I am really full, so thanks anyway but I am done!" We will spend some time talking a little about different food types, foods to avoid, the benefits of eating protein in weight loss. Most of the readers already know this so we will not waste fifty pages repeating what most of you know. Instead, let's focus on what I have called the "Ten Rules of Eating." These rules may seem so obvious that nutritional experts who write those four-hundred-page diet books will scorn and laugh. I say, "Let's make some simple life rules that actually work, and can be taught, embedded in your conscious life and allow you to transform your eating habits! These rules are not as much about what you eat but more about how much you eat, creating satiety (sense of feeling full) maintaining satiety without eating huge portions, and in general what I refer to as, *"connecting your brain to your mouth!"* These dietary rules are common sense, and are about 'moderation not elimination'!" If you adopt these rules, the average person will eliminate 1,000-2,000 calories a day from their intake of food, with any sense of deprivation. Following these rules can have an amazing effect. This is the equivalent of walking 3-5 hours a day on a treadmill. So take the rules seriously, embrace them and watch as you lose weight rather effortlessly.

Rule #1: If you are not hungry, don't eat!

It almost seems ridiculous to have to state this rule. However it is rule #1 for a very good reason. Almost every overweight adult breaks this rule repeatedly every day! You have had a pretty decent breakfast, some orange juice, and coffee and head off to work. You get to work and your co-worker says, "Hey John, someone just brought in donuts. Have a few!" You know that you are not hungry, but heck, it's free and I just love those Dunkin Donuts! So you eat two. That is 450 calories!

Later that day you have a good lunch. Then you realize that you are supposed to attend a meeting at 2:00 pm. You show up and the boss had them cater in some sandwiches, cookies, and soda. You are not hungry. But heck, it's free and who knows when you will get to dinner. So you have a sandwich, an oatmeal cookie and a Coke. That is another 550 calories. So by 2:00 pm this day you have already eaten about one third of a healthy caloric intake for the whole day, in addition to your usual breakfast and lunch, and at times when you were not even hungry. Many people just do this unconsciously. They do not think about the relationship between hunger and eating except when they are hungry. And of course when they are hungry they eat a lot! We will talk more about hunger and satiety (feeling full) later.

If you are going to get thin, or thinner, you must become aware of hunger, or the lack of hunger. When we dissociate hunger from eating behavior and eat reflexively, or as a means to relieve anxiety, depression or boredom, or just to be polite, we get fat. How often have you been at work, or at a friend's house and they offer some delectable, and usually high-calorie, treat. When offered this, almost every overweight adult accepts the offer and eats this food. This is a big problem.

So, it is critical that we begin to connect the sensation of hunger to eating. There will be no more eating when you are not hungry. No more, "I'm bored" eating, "Hey that looks delicious (even though I am not hungry)" eating, "watching TV" eating, "I am depressed" eating, "Aunt Maggie just brought an apple pie over (even though I am not hungry)" eating, "My boyfriend just broke up with me" eating, "I've got nothing else to do" eating, "Hey, it's a buffet, look at all that food" eating, "Wow, a free donut" eating, "I already ate lunch, but that looks good" eating, etc. etc. There is NO eating unless you are hungry. We are going to connect eating and putting food in your mouth, only when you have the sensation of hunger. Adopting this new approach to eating will probably cut out 800 calories a day from your eating. That is the equivalent of about 2 hours on a treadmill. Think about that every time you put something in your mouth when you are not hungry.

When you are not hungry it usually means that there is enough glucose in your bloodstream to tell your brain that you are not hungry. When we have plenty of fuel (glucose) in our bloodstream, we are already releasing insulin to store glucose as fat. When we eat again while we are releasing insulin, we just release another spike of insulin and nearly all of those extra 1,000 calories eaten when we were not hungry gets stored as fat.

So, the next time you get offered food when you are not hungry, just say NO. "Thanks for the offer. I love donuts, but I am not hungry." Now that wasn't so hard. You can do this. Let's connect hunger and eating. If you thought this rule was silly, here is rule #2.

Rule #2: When you are full, you're done!!

This also seems a little ridiculous. However it is rule #2 for a very good reason. It probably is the most important eating rule. Almost every overweight adult breaks this rule repeatedly every day. Why is this a huge problem, when it seems like such an obvious and logical eating rule? For many people it is related to what we have been taught during our childhood. This is particularly true for the baby boomers. Our parents often grew up on tight budgets. Food was valued highly. We would sit down to dinner and mom would bring out large portions for everyone. Your plate is full of food. Unfortunately, you were not even that hungry since you snuck a snack without mom knowing it half an hour ago.

Mom says, "I worked all afternoon preparing this meal, so I hope everyone enjoys it." Feeling guilty. You start eating even though you are not hungry (breaking Rule #1). After eating about a third of what mom gave you are totally full. You try to dish some off to the dog, but he is not hungry and won't eat it! Mom says. "Frank, you have hardly touched your food. I want you to clean your plate." Feeling guilty again. "OK, Mom." So you keep eating. Your stomach is about to burst and you finally nearly finish it. "Good job Frank. You cleared your plate." This is powerful positive reinforcement for stuffing food in our stomach long after we are full. This is how we create fat kids and overweight adults. Much more about this in Chapter Eight.

Now you are an overweight adult, struggling with your weight problems. You go out to a restaurant with some friends. You have a cocktail. You look at the menu. You are hungry. Everything on the menu looks great. You order a salad to be "healthy," and an entre' which comes with a baked potato, and two other side dishes. The portions are huge at this restaurant. That is why you love it. It is a good value. You get about 3,000 calories in a dinner for only $12. What a deal.

You eat the salad, which you ordered with blue cheese dressing and extra dressing on the side. You have already had two dinner rolls with large portions of butter. The other thing that you love about this restaurant is that the service is fast. You have barely finished your salad with extra dressing and two rolls (total of about 1,400 calories so far). Before you can absorb this large caloric bolus, and begin to raise your blood glucose level, you start digging into your steak, with baked potato and two other butter-drenched vegetables. The steak is a huge 16-ounce porterhouse, which is your favorite. Even though you have eaten too much food, the wrong kinds of food and eaten too fast (see Rule #8), you are still feeling pretty full after finishing less than half of your entre'. However, ever aware in your subconscious mind of the evils of wasting food, you keep eating, and eating. You finish the steak, the baked potato with butter and sour cream, of course, and even most of the butter soaked vegetables. You have just eaten another 2,000 calories, and at least half of those were eaten after you were well past the point of feeling full. If we add this to the extra 1,000 calories that you ate earlier in the day when you were not hungry, we have already eaten more than 2,000 excess calories in one day that you ate when you were either not hungry, or full. And then we wonder why we can't lose weight even though we walked for 45 minutes on the treadmill that morning (see Chapter Four).

We must stop eating past the point of full. Some of the rules to follow are going to repeatedly refer back to this critical Rule #2. There are many ways that we can adaptively make ourselves full or satiated. However, these tips and rules will only work if we totally ingrain rule #2. You must not eat any more food once you are full. Push the plate away and send it back to the kitchen. I doubt that you are going to FedEx the food in a container to a hungry child in a third world country. So you can choose. This excess food can either go in the garbage, in a doggy bag, or in your fat cells. I repeat, when you are full you are DONE! My ten-year-old daughter has this rule down cold. She used to feel obliged to try to finish her food. Now she often stops after eating less than a quarter of her dinner. She says. "Dad, I am full, so I'm done." She will not be an overweight adult. Her favorite rule, however, is the next rule.

Rule #3: Dessert is not a reward for breaking Rule #2!

Pretty funny huh? Actually, it is not so funny that we have become a culture of the sweet tooth. We have grown up being told that if we clear our plate, we can have dessert. Let's think about what horrible and distorted eating messaging many of us have grown up with. We start out eating a dinner when we are not hungry. We eat half of our meal and we are told we must keep eating even though we are full. Now we have made things even more maladaptive by being told that our prize for doing breaking the two fundamental, and common sense eating rules is to get a huge, sweet dessert as the reward. No wonder 70% of adults are overweight. We have been programmed so badly. We have disconnected eating from our conscious mind.

I do not think that we need or should have a dessert with every meal. At one point in my life I actually used to have a dessert after breakfast. I cannot really imagine that now. However, unlike most other diet books you will read, I am going to say that a small sweet dessert, of just about anything you like, at the end of your dinner is OK. Obviously, having a big dessert 3-4 times per day is going to disrupt the eating goals for any weight loss plan.

If you have carefully followed rules 1 and 2, as above, and you are not completely full, it is OK to save a little room for a small sweet dessert at the end of dinner. We are not talking about a 5 inch wide piece of chocolate cake or a 4-scoop hot fudge sundae. We are talking about a small dessert. Maybe a couple of bites of cake, or a few bites of a crème brule', etc. We are talking about 100 calories worth of dessert, not 1,200 calories of dessert. We are talking about having three bites, not three cookies.

I do support and agree with the usual diet book teaching that a little bit of fruit, or a small portion of sorbet which is fat free is better than even a small portion of that awesome cake. But, this book is about moderation, not complete deprivation. If you are following the other rules, and you are doing the work to change your metabolic rate, you deserve a small (dessert) reward occasionally. When you get really fit, and achieve your ideal fit and lean body weight, there may even come a time when you will need to eat a little more sweets so you don't lose weight. This is really possible. Also remember that if you are full you are done, so skip the dessert. Dessert is not a reward for eating past the point of full.

Rule #4: Protein, protein, protein. Atkins was (partially) right

I am not going to spend thirty to fifty pages outlining the "Atkin's" diet. I presume that just about every person who is reading this book has heard of Atkins. Atkins made a very important observation about the relationship between carbohydrate intake and weight gain, and loss. Atkins was one of the first to really promote high protein intake and the near elimination of carbohydrates from the adult diet in order to lose weight. It works. And, Atkins was partially right.

Protein diets are highly effective in promoting weight loss. If you remember the earlier chapter, we discussed the virtues of protein rather than carbohydrate and fats in our diet. First, the body cannot quickly or easily convert proteins into glucose. This conversion takes energy and time. Thus, after a protein-based meal one does not get nearly as large of an insulin spike to convert glucose to fat. Second, protein is broken down into amino acids, which are shipped to your cells to make proteins in, and on the surface of your cells. These amino acids are also crucial to the building and/or rebuilding and remodeling of skeletal muscle after you have stressed you muscles with the Burn Calories workout, crunches in your car and with isometric fidgeting.

Finally, when protein does get converted to glucose it happens slowly. When glucose levels go up slowly, it dramatically reduces the insulin spikes that are responsible for major fat storage and the precursor to type 2 diabetes. Glucose produced from the conversion of protein also is more of a sustained release from of glucose. As a result, the feeling of satiety and the curbing that hunger is longer lasting. This sustained satiety effect is much better than the rapid release and clearance of glucose after large insulin spikes that occur in a short time frame after a refined carbohydrate load, leading some people to talk about rebound hunger after eating refined carbohydrates.

Remember that I said Atkins was partially right. Where was he off track? He basically said that as long as you avoided or eliminated carbohydrates, eating protein, including protein containing very high fat content (like a fatty rib eye steak) was just fine. He also allowed a lot of egg consumption, with the high cholesterol loads associated with egg yolks. The Atkins approach would condone putting a lot of butter on protein based foods, or complex carbohydrates. He did not really adequately warn people away from the fat content associated with some forms of protein. He also failed to recognize that some modest intake of complex carbohydrates, especially in grazing mode or as a small snack one-half hour before a planned meal, will help a lot in getting a sense of satiety, or feeling full. This will, in turn, promote a decrease in total caloric intake for most individuals. I prefer and recommend what many might call a modified Atkins approach. Dr. Dean Ornish is one of the world leaders in creating a healthy and sustainable eating plan. His approach is endorsed in this book and is far superior to an Atkins approach. The Ornish philosophy about eating a healthy diet is summarized, by Dr. Ornish himself, later in this chapter.

Here are some great tips about a modified Atkins approach to eating that is healthy and sustainable. First, I agree with Atkins that we should eat a lot of protein and drink a lot of water. The best forms of protein would include lean meat and fish, and vegetable-based proteins, assuming that you can tolerate them. If you are a vegetarian, you are probably not reading this book because you have pretty good weight control already. If you are a vegetarian, or want to be a vegetarian it is still possible to create a high protein content diet. I would refer you to a myriad of diet books and cookbooks that will give you dozens if not hundreds of specific suggestions about high protein vegetarian options. This book provides a guide to eating, but it is not a cookbook.

Whether you are vegetarian or a carnivore it will be very important that you avoid the (bad), high fat content that is associated with some forms of (good) protein. Here are a few examples. Substitute a very lean filet mignon for a fatty rib eye or NY strip steak. Eat white meat chicken without the skin rather than a drumstick (dark meat) with the skin. These types of modifications of a high protein diet will dramatically reduce the fat and calorie content of an Atkin's approach to eating.

Eat eggs. When you eat eggs put in 3 egg whites with one yolk. This tastes great and similar to 3 eggs with 3 yolks. It has that yellow color, but has one third of the cholesterol. It is a very pure form of protein. Next, do not cook that omelet in 2 tablespoons of butter. Use a small amount of poly-unsaturated vegetable oil, or olive oil, rather than butter. Eat hard-boiled eggs or egg salad, but again eat less or none of the yolk which contains the high levels of cholesterol (see Chapter Six).

Use Smart One butter substitutes, and those with omega-3 fatty acids (fish oils). Eat fish, but in moderation in consideration of the source, and avoiding high levels or mercury associated with some ocean and river species. Do not eat fried fish (i.e., fish and chips) and then say to your wife, "See how healthy I am eating. I had fish for lunch." Yeah, and in that fried batter, you also had about 1,000 calories of fat and processed carbohydrates. You might as well have had a cheeseburger. It might have been lower in calories and with less fat and more protein than the fish and chips.

There are also some very high quality protein supplements, made by numerous companies. Some of the best powders contain vegetable based proteins like whey protein. If you find it palatable, make yourself a smoothie with these protein drinks or powders, combined with some blended fresh fruits or vegetables, mixed with low fat or fat free milk or possibly fruit juice. Mix it with skim milk and frozen berries. This is healthy, relatively low calorie, and will suppress your hunger for a longer period than a donut will. The protein may also enhance muscle remodeling and growth of lean muscle mass.

So, in summary, Atkins was partially right. Protein is a great food source to increase and sustain satiety, lower insulin spiking, and to provide amino acid substrate to build actively metabolizing skeletal muscle. However, a pure protein diet is not healthy. Some carbohydrate will help curb appetite, even though protein is better at sustaining satiety. We also need vitamins, healthy oils (like fish oils and some unsaturated vegetable oils, like safflower or olive oil), and complex carbohydrates, including fresh grains, etc, as outlined by Dr. Ornish. We need to avoid high cholesterol and high fat intake, which raises serum cholesterol, and triglycerides and promotes weight gain (fats have incredibly dense calorie content) and vascular disease (atherosclerosis). This is the bottom line. Protein, protein, protein is right, but one should balance this with healthy fresh complex carbohydrates (fruits and vegetables) and some healthy fats. It is also healthy to drink a lot of water every day to promote kidney health and protein metabolism. We have already touched on many of the issues related to the next rule. This next rule is a continuation of the modified Atkins/high protein approach to modifying our eating.

RULE #5: AVOID FATS, FRIED FOODS, AND (REFINED) CARBOHYDRATES (ESPECIALLY BEFORE BEDTIME)

It is almost cruel. We are genetically programmed to desire and love foods with very high caloric density. Fatty foods, fried and fatty foods, sugar and sweet carbohydrate foods are just about every American's favorite. Let's face it. For most people there is nothing better than a mouthwatering large, juicy, cheeseburger on a huge white bread bun, with super-sized French fries, and finished off with a creamy chocolate milkshake. We are talking about 3,000 calories just for lunch here.

Americans and most humans love these fatty foods, and foods with high content of processed carbohydrates, including chocolate cake, cupcakes, ice cream, chocolate chip cookies, cheesecake, etc. It is hard to completely eliminate the craving and consumption of these "to be avoided" foods. However, there are a number of tricks, in addition to following the "10 Rules" that will allow you to substantially reduce your consumption of the bad processed carbohydrates and fats in your diet. Notice that this rule is about avoiding and modulating fat and carbohydrate intake. Unlike many fad diets I am not forcing you to completely eliminate all of this from your diet. This is about moderation and modulation, not total deprivation and elimination. This is why these rules are sustainable.

So, here are some additional pearls of wisdom to allow you to eat some of the foods that you love or even crave, and still greatly reduce daily caloric intake and lose weight. If you eat a sandwich, or a hamburger (not forbidden under my dietary and cholesterol management rules), take half the bread off before eating it! Use a fork and knife to eat your hamburger with half the bun. This just took 120 calories or highly processed carbohydrate out of the hamburger meal. If you are having a tuna melt or a chicken salad sandwich, or any other sandwich, again, take off half of the bread and save 100 calories.

If you want a chocolate chip cookie for desert because you have not eaten past full and have a craving for some desert, do this. Take the cookie, break it in half and throw half into the garbage can. Then slowly eat the remaining half of a cookie. Now you have created a low(er) calorie desert (110 calories instead of 220 calories). And, once you start doing these tricks, you will notice two things: 1.) you do not really notice the difference between a half of a cookie and a whole one and 2.) You are losing weight! You will notice the difference when you get on the scale after a year of modifying your eating habits in this way

Ok, you like potato chips. So do I. Not great. This is a processed and fatty and high calorie content carbohydrate. What do you do? Open the bag and before you start your meal, throw 1/3 to 1/2 of the chips in the garbage can. This just gave you a bag of potato chips with half the calories. If you eat slowly, you will get satiated and you will not miss those extra chips. Use this same trick with French fries! Yes, I eat at McDonalds on occasion. I am not recommending that anyone eat fast food, but... I do love their French fries. I take half the order and throw it in the garbage before I sit down to eat. Eat slowly. Do these (half) maneuvers on a regular basis and you will not notice the difference except in your waist size a year later. It really adds up.

Use low calorie vinaigrette dressing rather than fat and mayonnaise-based dressings (thousand island, blue cheese, etc.) on your salad. One of the occult abuses of the diet conscious American adult is to have a beautiful salad with all of those wonderful and healthy fresh vegetables, like tomatoes, green peppers, carrots, etc. They add great protein, with strips of white meat chicken that is not deep-fried in carbohydrate batter. But then, they put six ounces of Thousand Island dressing on this salad, adding nearly 1,000 calories of fat onto this otherwise great, high fiber, vitamin and protein-rich meal. Stop that. Use a smaller serving of a low fat balsamic vinaigrette dressing. Then you will have all of the good things (protein, complex antioxidants, complex carbohydrates vegetables, vitamins, etc.) but with 700 calories less fat content. When you make these adjustments, it will make a difference. Remember two plus two equals four. You must combine good eating with good burning to become thin and fit.

You love ice cream. So do I. This is one of the highest fat content foods in the world, besides pure lard. Can you eat ice cream? Better not to, but if you do let's modulate this. Rather than a three scoop, banana split with eight ounces of whip cream, and three sauces, etc. (about 1,200 calories), let's eat slowly and downsize this to a very small scoop (children's portion) with a small portion of hot fudge or caramel in a sundae (300 calories). Let's be even better. Take two-teaspoon bites from your daughter's small sundae! This is called moderation, not elimination. Of course, elimination is better. You are full after eating your dinner and you say "I am full so I am done. No dessert for me this evening, thanks. Let's have the check and go home." Now you are really getting and living the "Rules."

Finally, eating food in general and especially fatty or carbohydrates late at night and before you go to sleep is one of the worst abuses of this rule. If you eat a piece of cake, a brownie, a cookie or ice cream shortly before you go to sleep, this will trigger an insulin spike at absolutely the worst time. You are about to sleep and go into a low metabolic need state. So, when you eat that snack before bedtime and then release a spike of insulin, virtually all of these excess calories get stored as fat. There is a book written several years ago entitled, "No White at Night," that really focused on this key rule of no carbohydrates later in the day. This is right on. Avoid these late night snacks, keep insulin levels low when you head off to sleep, and stop pouring those calories into fat cells.

Rule #6: Grazing. Many Small Meals Each Day

We have raised the issue of insulin spikes many times in the book. Insulin is evil for adults that want to be thin and fit, and not diabetic. How can we reduce these evil insulin spikes? We can eat the right kind of foods (i.e., Rules #4 and 5). We can also eat small meals, 4-6 times per day rather than eating two or three massive meals per day. This habit of eating small amounts throughout the day to suppress your hunger with the potential to reduce your total caloric intake has been referred to as grazing. Grazing is what many wild animals do, particularly herbivores. Have you ever seen an obese horse or giraffe? No. You have not seen this because these animals graze (eat small amounts at frequent intervals) and eat protein and complex carbohydrates, rather than eating two or three massive, fat and carbohydrate loaded meals a day.

If humans follow the behavior of these types of mammals they will be thin, regardless of the genetics that they are born with. Small, low carbohydrate content snacks and meals will keep insulin spiking to a minimum. The glucose that is made available in your bloodstream will be diverted to your skeletal muscle, brain, heart, etc. where it is needed for energy and cell maintenance. There will be very little leftover glucose, and very little insulin to instruct your body to take all of this glucose and send it to your fat cells to make triglycerides and more fat.

If you don't graze, and go for 4-5 hours without eating, you will probably be starving when you finally sit down to your lunch or dinner. Many overweight adults let themselves get this hungry. They are ravenous. They sit down to their lunch or dinner, ready to really dig in. They are in a hurry because either have a short lunch break or they have to run to the store or pick up the kids, so now you are starving and in a hurry. What do you do? You sit down, and eat a lot of food—very fast. Maybe you gorge down 3,000 calories in 10-15 minutes. You eat so much, so fast that your brain and stomach never even have the time to send a signal to your primitive brain that glucose is plentiful, and you can slow down and stop eating. Fifteen minutes after you have ingested your entire caloric allowance for the day, you feel really full. It is too late. The horse is out of the barn. You have not technically broken rule #2 because you ate so much, so fast. Unfortunately you are on the wide road to obesity. This massive and fast eating 2-3 times per day has to stop if you want to get "thin" or thinner. We will focus again on the key concept of eating slowly in Rule #8.

The other critical issue related to smaller portions and smaller meals relates to stomach size and satiety. The two key signals to the brain to tell you that you are full are 1) increases in blood glucose level, and 2) distention of the stomach which releases hormones and transmits nerve signals to the brain to tell you that you are full. If you chronically (for years and years) eat very large meals 2-3 times a day, rather than small portions 5-6 times a day, there is evidence that your stomach will enlarge over time. When this happens you need larger and larger portions to feel full, so you end up never feeling satiated unless you eat huge portions ("the more you eat the more you will eat!"). This creates this vicious circle so it feeds into the corollary of this observation, which is, "the fatter you get, the fatter you get."

The less you eat, the less you will eat

BURN CALORIES WHILE YOU SLEEP – TIM A. FISCHELL M.D.

This question has been looked at scientifically by inflating balloons in the stomach and measuring the size of the stomach in obese individuals. The stomach does grow over time with large portions in obese people. Conversely, the stomach capacity can decrease after a restrictive diet in obese adults. This is great news. If you start eating smaller portions, and eating slowly your stomach can get smaller and you will begin to feel full with less food and without major bariatric surgery to surgically reduce the size of your stomach. This now creates the equally important observation in people who will follow the eating rules. When you eat small portions (graze) and you eat slowly and you follow rule #8, which will help you be able to follow these other rules, you will also find that the other important corollary about grazing which is, "The less you eat, the less you will eat." This is critical. As you eat less and smaller portions throughout the day, you will have less hunger, your stomach will remodel and shrink over time. After several years of adopting these healthy eating rules you will not be able to tolerate, or even imagine eating the large portions that you are eating today. You will be too full to eat it because your stomach will be smaller, and distended with small portions rather than huge portions. You will be full with much less food, and you will follow Rule #2!

So, grazing, or the habit of having smaller meals more frequently is a great way to attack your weight problems. There is another variation of this grazing technique. Rule #7 outlines a great trick to create satiety, suppress your hunger, and eliminate that ravenous craving to eat a massive dinner.

RULE # 7: EAT A SMALL SNACK ½ HOUR BEFORE DINNER (YOUR MOTHER WAS RIGHT!)

There are two key signals to your brain that tell you that you are full. The first key signal is the amount of glucose in your bloodstream. When you eat a lot of food or especially sweets, high sugar content and processed carbohydrates, your blood glucose will go up. This triggers the release of insulin, which instructs your body to store the glucose as fat, mainly by producing triglycerides. It also has bad effects in producing higher levels of cholesterol. We will talk much more about cholesterol in Chapter Seven.

Rising blood glucose also triggers the release of other chemicals including a hormone called leptin that sends a signal to your brain that you are full. The main thrust of this rule is to get you to get into the habit of having a small appetizer, such as a complex carbohydrate snack about half an hour before your big meal of the day. The insulin released from a small carbohydrate snack, combined with the effect of insulin promotes the entry of tryptophan into your brain and thereby produces another key brain neurotransmitter, serotonin. Serotonin can enhance mood and suppress hunger. The production of serotonin by the ingestion of carbohydrate and insulin release may explain why some overweight individuals crave carbohydrates.

Eating some form of low glycemic carbohydrate, such as lentils, beans, whole grains, and high fiber foods may be an optimal source of carbohydrates to suppress your appetite half an hour before a planned meal. This will raise your blood glucose level, and your brain serotonin level, just prior to your biggest meal of the day (usually dinner).

You may say, "But that will ruin my ability to gorge out and to eat my whole dinner!" Exactly. Your mother was right. That snack before dinner will ruin your appetite. This is the whole point of Rule #7. I want you to eat less food, without feeling starved or deprived. That is what this rule is about.

So, now you know what to do. Eat a small snack before dinner. Your blood sugar rises. You begin dinner with a relatively high level of satiety. Then, you sit down to that huge dinner and you can only eat about one third of the dinner before you are completely full. Stop eating now! Remember, the critical Rule #2, "When you are full, you are done."

Some people may call this wasteful. I call it getting thin! If you are worried about wasting food, I have a few solutions. First, prepare smaller portions. The less you eat the less you will eat. Next, save the food as leftovers, if you liked it and you are thrifty.

Do NOT however break Rule #2. Eat a snack, then eat dinner, and when you are full you are done. You are now heading in the direction of thin.

Rule # 8: Eat slowly!

This is a key rule as well. This is another variation of Rules 6 and 7 (grazing and snacking before dinner to ruin your appetite). It is about creating and maintaining a state of satiety in order to reduce our daily caloric intake, eliminate massive ingestion of food that leads to insulin spiking, and accomplishing this without feeling deprived or hungry.

At different times in our lives, we had to grab food "on the run." When I was an intern in internal medicine and on call in the hospital, my pager was going off for some crisis every 4-5 minutes. We would have a free, house staff dinner in the cafeteria served between 8:00 p.m. and 10:00 p.m. If you did not show up then, you probably would not get to eat that night, other than getting a Twinkie out of a vending machine. As my pager would go off three times in ten minutes, I learned quickly to load up my plate, and gorge, 3,000 calories in six minutes. Luckily, I was young and thin and so busy and metabolically "burning" calories that this highly maladaptive habit did not make me fat. If I did the same thing today, even with my commitment to exercising, there would be serious consequences in terms of weight gain.

Eating a lot of food very fast is bad. Americans eat too fast. We like fast food and fast service. We are on the run and need to grab a meal and often eat like the on-call intern. The problem with this is this leads us to eat too much. The calories are ingested before our closed-loop feedback that tells us that we have eaten enough. We do not have a chance to feel satiety before the bad deed (overeating) is history.

The next section talks a little more about the key satiety signals to our brain. These are the signals that tell us that we are full. After eating even high carbohydrate loaded foods, there is a "lag" or "hysteresis," in feeling the effect of this caloric load. This means that you will eat the 3,000 calories in ten minutes, but it will take another ten to fifteen minutes for the satiety signals of rising blood glucose or stomach distention to tell your primitive brain that you are full. Since you do not get this signal until it is too late to feel full you may be able to stuff away 3,000 calories without breaking Rule #2.

The critical message here is that we need to eat slowly, so that our nervous system and blood sugar levels can begin to tell us that we are satiated before we have eaten too much food. If we eat slowly, taking at least 30-40 minutes to eat our meals, then we will have time to get that signal telling our brain, "I am full." Then if we follow Rule #2, we will be done, before the 3,000 calories in front of us have been eaten and before they are speeding to fill our fat cells after a huge insulin spike. Eat slowly. Then stop eating when you feel full (Rule #2) and start to get control of your overeating. This is common sense, simple and effective.

RULE # 9: NO SUGARED DRINKS!

This rule does not apply to everyone. If you do not consume sugared drinks you can skip this rule. However, there are a lot of overweight adults who just love their soda or "pop." This is a huge industry in the United States. Just look at the commercials during the Super Bowl and you will get that Americans drink a lot of Coke and Pepsi.

These sugared drinks which include Coca Cola, Pepsi, Root Beer, Dr. Pepper, Seven-up, etc., etc., are basically flavored and carbonated sugar drinks with virtually no nutritional value. These drinks are essentially pure sugar (processed carbohydrates) non-nutritional, high caloric, and a waste of calories. One can of regular soda will typically contain 110-130 calories of sugar. Many individuals think nothing about drinking four to five of these a day. For an average, sedentary middle-aged adult that would represent nearly 25% of the entire prescribed caloric content of a day in order to be in "weight neutral" eating. To burn off those "sugared drinks" it would take almost two hours of walking on a treadmill. That is a lot of wasted and totally "empty" calories. Not only do these drinks promote insulin release and storage of this rapidly absorbed bolus of sugar into fat, recent studies demonstrate that drinking these sugared drinks also have an independent and potent effect in raising blood pressure. A recent study conducted in Great Britain and the U.S. (INTERMAP Study) showed a very significant correlation between sugared drink intake and high blood pressure, with an average of 1.6 mm Hg increase in systolic blood pressure for every one sugared drink per day. This is important, and is enough to contribute to a higher risk of stroke and heart attack in those individuals who consume two to three or more sugared drinks per day. In contrast to sugared drinks, diet sodas showed no associated high blood pressure risk.

This may be a tough habit to break if you love your pop, as they call it in the Midwest. However, it is one of the easier ways to really reduce or eliminate wasted and non-nutritional caloric intake if you are an individual that loves these drinks.

How about substituting diet soft drinks instead? Many health experts are really down on the diet drinks. These drinks have substituted additives like aspartame or saccharin for sugar. Are these bad for you? Probably not too bad in moderation. That is, if you are trying to lose weight, and you love these sodas or other sugared drinks, in the long run it is probably much healthier to substitute the diet drink for the sugared one. This may eliminate

400-500 calories a day from your intake. These diet drinks are probably safe in moderation. If you have two or three per day this is likely to be very safe. If you have ten a day we know less about the long-term effects. The bottom line is soda and carbonated sugared drinks are bad. Diet sodas are less bad and can be consumed in moderation. If you do not drink them at all and drink bottled water or vitamin water this is even better.

How about healthier drinks that contain sugar like fruit juice? Most fruit juices are also relatively high in sugar and calories. However, certain unsweetened fruit juices may be OK in moderation. I happen to love orange juice, especially fresh-squeezed. This contains a lot of Vitamin C, which is a great vitamin to enhance your immune system, help build connective tissue and repair minor injuries in your ligaments, tendons, and muscle. Other juices have key vitamins as well and unlike soda, may have some nutritional and medicinal value. So, my advice is fresh fruit juice in moderation, but let's stop with the pop!

Rule # 10: Alcohol in moderation

Alcohol is good for you, as long as it is done in moderation. Studies have shown that drinking a relatively small amount of alcohol every day will raise your good cholesterol and will prolong your life.

Remember that I said "in moderation." This means about one or two drinks per day, at most, for women and two to three drinks per day, at most for men. If a little is good maybe more is better? Not! Alcohol consumption that exceeds these guidelines is not good for you or for your diet. Imagine being meticulous about following rules 1-9. This is great. Then you get home and tell the wife that you are going out with the guys for a few drinks. Americans also love their beer. So after a great day of following the rules and having moderation and satiety and ingesting only 2,400 calories which puts you on the path to thin, you go out for a few beers with the guys. This turns out to be six beers with the guys! This is another 800 calories of carbohydrates, carbohydrates at night before you go to bed (insulin spiking at low activity time = FAT). Stop this behavior. Drink in moderation. Raise your HDL (good cholesterol, and follow Rule #10). OK, a couple of times a year it is fun to party. You have permission, but not every week— and certainly not every day.

Now that you know the ten critical rules to eating to get thin, let's emphasize a few other key concepts about eating and weight loss.

AMERICANS AND THEIR RESTAURANTS

Let's face it, Americans love to eat and they love a good deal. What could be a better deal than fast food? Almost all fast food chains have three things in common. First, they serve it fast so we can eat a lot of calories in a short time and break Rule # 8. In addition, you can get a lot of calories for very little money; the food they have created is tasty and fulfills our genetic cravings for fatty and high calorie content foods, and Remember, feast or famine from Chapter One. Unfortunately, this has been particularly troublesome and maladaptive for poorer Americans, who legitimately may feel that they want to get a lot of food for little money. It also explains why there is a relationship between lower incomes and obesity. Less well-off Americans tend to favor high calorie content foods, as a cost savings maneuver. You can buy a lot of calories at McDonald's or Wendy's or KFC for very little money. Unfortunately, it is also a health-destroying maneuver.

Some of the most popular non-fast food restaurants (like Denny's, Big Boy, Olive Garden, etc.) are also well known for creating very high caloric meals at reasonable prices. The average American wants to get a good value, so he or she loves it when they dish out a huge portion, filling every square inch of the dinner plate with a huge slab of fried meat, three vegetables (fried of course) along with three rolls, a salad with fatty dressing and ½ price for dessert with the entre special. He thinks to himself, "Wow, this is the best restaurant ever. Did you see how much food I just got for $12.95? And on Wednesdays, the kids' get about the same portion for half price. What a deal!" (I ate well. I had fish—

yeah, fish and chips and grease). Even better are those all-you-can-eat specials or buffets. This is a super favorite of super-sized adults.

Other hidden amazing facts include some of the massive caloric content in some foods. I had dinner the other day at the Cheesecake Factory. The food there is good, but the portions are ridiculously large in most cases. I was curious about their cheesecake (I like cheesecake) and said, "That must be incredibly high in calories." The waitress told me, "Yes, the full slice of cheesecake is about 1,200 calories, but that is not the worst dessert." I asked her, "What could be more caloric than cheesecake?" She tells me that one piece of the carrot cake is 2,400 calories. Wow. That is close to the entire day's recommended caloric intake for most adults. Amazingly, some people think nothing of finishing off their 2,500 calorie large portion meal there with a 2,400 piece of carrot cake. That is 4,900 calories, and that was just their dinner. These same folks will say, "But doctor, I don't really eat that much."

Overweight people are very good at kidding themselves, and grossly underestimating how much they eat and the caloric content of what they eat. I do not want you to count, and diary your calories, but you must be aware of the caloric content of food, and follow the eating rules, and tips. People who frequent these all-you-can-eat restaurants, or buffets, ignore the caloric content and portion sizes of what they eat, and ignore the eating rules of Chapter Five will be eating their way to be a contestant on the Biggest Loser. You need to connect your brain (satiety) to your mouth!

FOOD SUPPLEMENTS

We will talk a little more about this in the fad diets section in Chapter Six. There are some supplements that can make sense and be incorporated into you overall weight loss and fitness program. For example, there are some excellent protein-based powders. If you go into your local GNC store or most other "health food" stores, you may find more than a hundred of these protein supplements. The best of these are generally, vegetable-based (whey and soy), nearly pure protein and contain minimal fats or carbohydrate. This type of protein powder, can be mixed with a little milk, or fruit juice and/or other fresh fruits and vegetables, and then blended like a milkshake. This is a great snack or small meal for "grazing" and is also a great snack for Rule #7 (a small healthy "snack" a half hour before lunch or dinner). This is low calorie and high protein and will suppress hunger. This is a great pearl. As for other fat-burning supplements, these are scientifically unproven, expensive and probably of little or no value (see Chapter Six.)

Weigh Yourself Every Day! (Closing the Loop)

Most overweight adults do not want to step on a scale. They are afraid to see reality in the form of a cold, hard number on a digital display. This number is scary, and it is the result of decades of abuse of their body by a sedentary lifestyle, and by repeated violations of the eating rules outlined in this chapter.

These same individuals actually have a pretty good idea about how much they weigh. They just do not want to see it read 267 pounds (man) or 185 pounds (woman). OK, now let's chill about this number. You have to have a starting point. If you were not having troubles with weight and fitness you would not be reading this. As Mark Twain said, "I feel sorry for the poor bastards who do not have any vices. What are they going to give up when they get sick?"

If you did not need some friendly advice and some great tips about achieving health and fitness and weight loss, you would have already sold or given this book to a friend. It is time to get on the scale. Here is the good news. Once you initiate this program, start the Burn Calories workouts and follow the eating rules; you should never see a number this big on your scale again.

Why do I want you to weigh yourself every day? This is called closing the loop. In all electronic or mechanical or biological systems there are feedback loop controls. When the water gets too high, it spills over the dam, keeping the water level from getting too high. When the living room heats up on a super-hot summer day, the thermostat senses it, kicks on the air conditioning and cools the room (closed loop)! If no one is watching and there is no closed-loop control, things, like obesity, can get out of control. Eventually it gets to the point where reversing the problem just gets harder and harder, people give up all hope and have to just face the morbidity and mortality of their obesity. We do not want to go there.

This is why it is important to weigh yourself every day. Since there is a fair amount of weight variation based on the water content of your body, it is probably best to weigh yourself at about the same time every day. Morning will be less discouraging since you will be a little less hydrated and you will weigh a few pounds less than at night, but in the end it does not really matter. If you have been well behaved, and are burning calories and following the eating rules your weight will decline over time. I do not expect or want, "The Biggest Loser" kind of weight loss that you may see on TV. We are looking to achieve sustainable weight loss of about 2-4 pounds per week. That will be about 10-15 pounds of weight loss per month until you get to your plateau weight for the amount of effort that you are willing to put into the program. You could then choose to crank up the intensity on either the eating or burning (working out) side and set a new plateau weight target.

Other ways that you can close the loop include what some of my women friends call the "jean test." This means if your jeans are tight then you are putting on weight. This is better than nothing, but my goal is to have you achieve a new jean test. In this test, your jeans are so loose you need to head to the Gap or Old Navy because you have lost so much weight that your clothes don't fit anymore. Once you get to your target weight and you are happy, then you should either use the scale or the tight jean test to make sure that you are not re-gaining the weight.

How low can you go with your targeted weight? This is a very important question. Here is the main question I will ask you. What is the least you have weighed as an adult? This would not include any unusual situation like being in a coma with intravenous feeding for a year. If you are a man and weighed 176 pounds at age 21 and now you are at 245 pounds, you can get back to 176 pounds. You may have trouble believing it, and your friends may not recognize you, but you can get to this weight with focus and a plan that controls eating behavior and allow you to regain your skeletal muscle mass, and a youthful metabolic rate. If you do not close the loop by weighing yourself you probably have little chance of ever getting half of the way to that goal. This takes discipline, and loop-closing conscious feedback to your eating and working out behavior.

So now you are weighing yourself every morning. If you have gained a pound or two over two to three days, you'll need to make adjustments for the next several days to get back on track. This means more intensive following of the eating rules, and/or more crunches in your car, isometric fidgeting or maybe four workouts this week rather than three. If you do not weigh yourself, however, you are driving in the dark, and without headlamps! You need to close the loop, and adjust your behaviors on a daily basis to reach your weight and fitness goals.

SATIETY (FEELING FULL): THE LESS YOU EAT, THE LESS YOU'LL EAT

There are two key signals to your brain that tell you that you are full. The first key signal is the amount of glucose in your bloodstream. We have already talked about this in Rule #7. We have already talked about how to use a small snack, such as a complex carbohydrate snack about half an hour before your big meal of the day, to help to raise your blood glucose level just prior to your biggest meal of the day (usually dinner).

The other key signal to your brain that you are "full" is a nerve output from your stomach, when it is distended with food. Nerve fibers from your stomach transmit data to your brain. In addition, the stomach and upper small intestine can release hormones that also wend key satiety signals to your brain. When

112

we eat massive quantities of food on a regular basis, our stomachs will adapt. The stomach will slowly stretch or grow over time. When you do this and your stomach at age 45 has 50% greater volume capacity than it did at when you were twenty years old, you now have to eat a lot more food to fill and distend this stomach before it sends out the key signal to your brain to tell you that you are full. This can also be reversed as you graze (Rule #6), eat smaller portions because you ruined your massive dinner due to a snack before dinner (Rule #7) and because you ate slowly and let your brain see the glucose levels go up before you ate that massive plate of food (Rule #8). As you adopt these rules, and eat smaller portions, your stomach will also begin to get smaller, just like your waistline. As a result, you will get full more quickly after eating smaller portions, due to the distention of your smaller and remodeled stomach. You will then eat even less as you follow Rule #2 and stop eating past the point of full.

I call this observation of eating small portions, grazing and slow eating leading to earlier satiety, the shrinking of the stomach, and the inability to comfortably eat massive portions, "The less you eat, the less you eat." It is real. When you follow these rules, create and listen to satiety signals, close the loop on the scale (see below), and follow the type of healthy eating outlined by Dr. Ornish, at the end of the chapter, you will like the result. The only bad news is that it will be time to buy a new wardrobe of clothes.

Your old clothes will not fit, as you have created a new body and a new life.

Conversely, the more you eat (and chronically distend and remodel the stomach to be too big) the more you will need to eat, in order to distend this huge stomach to get "full." After twenty-to-thirty years of huge portions, and massive overeating, the stomach may no longer be able to remodel to a smaller size. This is when one may require a surgeon's scalpel to literally cut away half or more of your stomach (gastric reduction surgery) in order to shrink it so you can feel full again and lose weight. So, the more you eat the more you will eat! The focus of this book and these eating rules is to stop this destructive and vicious over-eating process before you need dangerous surgical intervention to save your life from your overeating. You need to *get full, feel and stay full, and recognize full* if you hope to lose weight. When you eat when you are *not* hungry, and eat past full you are ignoring the two huge danger road signs on the highway to health and you will be heading off the cliff to obesity, and to a shortened life, and driving off the road to a potentially fatal crash.

The approach in this book is crucial. You can take it to another level by really eating better foods. There are some great mentors who can teach us how to eat *better* and to live a healthier lifestyle. I am delighted to have the input about healthy eating and lifestyle from my friend, Dr. Dean Ornish. Dr. Ornish is a world-leading expert in the area of healthy eating and living. In the next section, Dr. Ornish summarizes some of his key messages to people who want to eat and live healthier.

Dr. Dean Ornish's Approach to a Healthy Diet

The way of eating that I recommend is not a diet in the usual sense of the word. Why? Because if you go *on* a diet, sooner or later you're likely to go *off* it.

Diets are all about what you *can't* have and *must* do. I've learned that even more than losing weight, most people want to feel free and in control. This goes back to the first diet—when God said, "Don't eat the apple." That didn't go very well, and that was God talking.

Instead, if you see your food choices each day as part of a spectrum, then you're more likely to feel free and empowered. There's no diet to go on, so there's no diet to go off—you can't fail. The more you change, the more you improve and the better you feel.

And the better you feel, the more likely you are to continue healthy changes in your diet and lifestyle—not just to live longer, but also to feel better. Because the biological mechanisms that control our health are so dynamic, most people find that they feel so much better, so quickly, it reframes the reason for making diet and lifestyle changes from fear of dying (which is not sustainable) to joy of living (which is).

What matters most is your *overall* way of eating and living. In thirty-five years of medical research, my colleagues and I at the non-profit Preventive Medicine Research Institute found that the more people changed their diet and lifestyle, the more they improved in whatever we measured—at *any* age.

It's not all or nothing; you have a spectrum of choices. Foods aren't good or bad, but some are healthier for you than others. To the degree you move in a healthier direction, there is a corresponding benefit. I categorized foods from the most healthful (Group 1) to the least healthful (Group 5).

So, if you indulge yourself one day, eat healthier the next. If you forget to exercise or meditate one day, do a little more the next. You get the idea.

Let's say you want to lower your cholesterol level by 50 points or your blood pressure by 10 mm, or your blood sugar by 20 points. Begin by making moderate changes in your diet and check these again in a few weeks. If that degree of change was enough to accomplish your goals, great, you're there. If not, you can either make bigger changes or go on medication.

Now, if you're trying to reverse a life-threatening illness, then you'd be wise to eat on the healthiest end of the spectrum. You'll need to make bigger changes to reverse heart disease than if you're just trying to lose a few pounds—the ounce of prevention and the pound of cure.

It's not low-carb vs. low-fat. An optimal diet is low in unhealthful carbs (both sugar and other refined carbohydrates) *and* low in fat, especially saturated fats and trans fats; and low in red meat and processed foods. Trans fats increase the shelf life of food products, but decrease the shelf life of the people who eat them.

Also, what you *include* in your diet is as important as what you *exclude*—high in healthful carbs such as fruits, vegetables, whole grains, legumes, soy products in whole, unrefined forms, and fish such as salmon that are rich in nourishing omega-3 fatty acids. There are literally hundreds of thousands of health-enhancing substances in these foods. For example, foods such as blueberries, tea, and chocolate (in small quantities) promote neurogenesis, causing more brain cells to grow. And what's good for you is good for the planet.

Calories count—fat has 9 calories per gram, but protein and carbohydrates have only 4 calories per gram; so when you eat less fat, you consume fewer calories without consuming less food.

117

Also, it's easy to eat too many calories from sugar and other refined carbohydrates because they are so low in fiber that you can consume large amounts without getting full. Sugar gets absorbed so quickly that you get repeated insulin surges, which promotes type 2 diabetes and accelerates the conversion of calories into body fat.

Choose quality over quantity, and *eat mindfully* so you have more pleasure with fewer calories. If you can afford it, organic foods taste much better and they're better for you. Many people are surprised to find that foods that they thought they didn't like—such as broccoli—are really good when you eat the organic version of them. Avoid processed foods and focus on those in their natural form.

In thirty-five years of medical research conducted at the nonprofit Preventive Medicine Research Institute, which I founded, we have seen that patients who ate mostly plant-based meals, with dishes like black bean vegetarian chili and whole wheat penne pasta with roasted vegetables, achieved reversal of even severe coronary artery disease. They also engaged in moderate exercise and stress-management techniques, and participated in a support group.

The program also led to improved blood flow and significantly less inflammation, which matters because chronic inflammation is an underlying cause of heart disease and many forms of cancer. We found that this program may also slow, stop, or reverse the progression of early-stage prostate cancer, as well as reverse the progression of type 2 diabetes.

Also, we found that it changed gene expression in over five-hundred genes in just three months, "turning on" genes that protect against disease and "turning off" genes that promote breast cancer, prostate cancer, inflammation, and oxidative stress.

The program, too, has been associated with increased telomerase, which increases telomere length, the ends of our chromosomes that are thought to control how long we live (studies done in collaboration with Dr. Elizabeth Blackburn, who was awarded the Nobel Prize in Medicine in 2009 for discovering telomerase). As our telomeres get longer, our lives may get longer.

In a randomized controlled trial, patients on this lifestyle program lost an average of 24 pounds after one year and maintained a 12-pound weight loss after five years. The more closely the patients followed this program, the more improvement we measured—at any age. Over a thousand patients on this program in West Virginia, Pennsylvania, and Nebraska lost almost 8 percent of their BMI after one year. For more information, please go to www.ornish.com.

DEAN ORNISH, M.D.

CHAPTER FIVE

KEY RULES ABOUT FOOD AND EATING

1) If you are not hungry, don't eat.

2) When you are full, you're done.

3) Dessert is not a reward for breaking Rule #2.

4) Protein, protein, protein (Atkins was partially right).

5) Avoid fats, fried foods, and carbohydrates.

6) Grazing (many small meals).

7) Eat a small snack ½ hour before dinner (your mother was right).

8) Eat slowly.

9) No sugared drinks.

10) One (at most two) alcoholic drinks per day.

Chapters One through Five

Key Points Weight Loss Summary

1) Understand metabolism why your metabolism has changed (lost muscle).

2) Understand metabolism; what happens when you eat carbs or too much food.

3) Commit to 40 minutes of aerobic weight lifting workout 2-3 times/week!

4) Read and the re-read the rules of eating; imprint them in your brain.

5) Follow the rules. The closer you get the faster you will lose weight.

6) Weigh yourself every day. Close the loop.

7) Shrink your stomach! Small portions. The less you eat, the less you can eat!

8) A huge portion at a restaurant is not a "good deal!"

9) Be realistic about rate of weight loss. This is NOT the "Biggest Loser."

10) Inspire and teach others; pass it forward (especially to your children)!

11) Affirmation: You can get to your ideal body weight!

❧ Chapter Six ❧

Fad Diets, Fad Exercising, and Why This Does Not Work (for most people)

Americans love a quick fix. We all want something for nothing; a great bargain; the best in the world at rock bottom prices. We want to get thin quick. We want a pill that we take once a day that will make us look like a supermodel within thirty days. We want an abdominal exercise machine that will do all the work for us while we sit back and drink a milkshake. We want a great diet that makes us always feel full, deprives us of nothing but let's us lose 30 pounds in two weeks. When it comes to exercise, we want it to be fun and not last long, and a free massage at the end would be nice too. We often have unrealistic expectations about what we are capable of doing. We try it. It is too difficult and not sustainable. We quit and become cynical.

The fad industry has capitalized on all of these weaknesses of the American consumer. Just like the fast food chains, they know the buzzwords and the "ingredients" to get you to eat their "propaganda," watch their infomercial, and make three easy payments on your Visa card to a fat free life. These are some but certainly not all of the reasons that we have had an amazing proliferation of videos, books, infomercials, magazine ads, etc., all promoting the easy path to immediate weight loss and fitness. It is big business. The problem is that most of the time the American consumer is wasting his or her time and money for foods, diet plans and fitness plans that are not based upon science, and are not sustainable or realistic, and in some cases are frankly dangerous to one's health.

Fad diets typically promise they are easy to follow and require no exercise. A fad diet may restrict entire food groups, or over-emphasize a super-food. These diets may require the use of supplements, usually marketed by the diet company. These diets usually do not give you tools to deal with daily challenges, such as eating out, social occasions or simple cravings. Because you do not learn long-term strategies for weight management, you are likely to regain any weight you do lose within one to five years. Examples of fad diets are the acai berry diet, the grapefruit diet, the cabbage soup diet and the HCG diet. A diet does not have to be nutritionally unsound to be a fad, but many fad diets are based on myth, theory, and hype, rather than fact.

This book is not intended to critique in detail each and every fad diet, food supplement, and fad exercise program promoted in the last ten years. That would require a two-thousand-page book. Instead, I would like to review the schemes, limitations and risks of various types of fad programs. This chapter is intended to try to educate the reader as a consumer and allow you to have a Buyer Beware attitude about fad dieting and exercising.

As I have tried to emphasize in the forward, this book is not a fad book. This book is intended to be in line with the advice and recommendations of the American Heart Association, Centers for Disease Control and Harvard School of Public Health and other scientific and public health organizations. These groups have made statements that support the development of lifelong habits that help you achieve a healthy weight, rather than fad diets that promise instant results.

The program in this book is aligned with this concept. It is based upon evidence-based science (not fad claims), and upon dietary guidelines and exercise physiology that makes sense and are sustainable for a lifetime, not just for thirty days. Dietary recommendations such as those provided by real scientific experts, like the ones outlined by Dr. Dean Ornish are more proven and carry benefit.

In contrast, let's focus upon the basic themes and pitfalls of fad diets, and then fad exercise programs. Hopefully this will help the reader understand the appeal, but also the problems and limitations of many of these plans. In the end it will help to explain why these programs do not work for most people.

Fad Diets

In an effort to lose weight quickly and easily, many people try fad diets. These diets may seem to be effective in the beginning, but any weight you lose is likely to be regained. Some of these diets are also unhealthy and may lead to health consequences. These fad diets typically have at least three or four common themes or claims.

Almost all fad diets claim that they will lead to rapid weight loss. Some will claim that you can lose up to 20-30 pounds in 2-3 weeks. The truth is that the most weight a person can lose in a day is about a half-pound. If one loses more than that it is almost always just loss of water weight. This rate of weight loss (1/2 pound per day) is also not healthy or sustainable. In most cases this will require massive caloric restrictions. The caloric restriction to achieve this degree of weight loss will significantly exceed the 2005 Dietary Guidelines for Americans, which defines a reasonable dietary restriction as a calorie deficit of 500 to 1,000 calories per day. Some of the "fad" diets may lead to calorie restrictions of 1,500-2,000 calories per day. Programs that encourage you to fast or put you near starvation can lead to fatigue, irritability, nutritional deficiencies and weakness. For example, the

Master Cleanse, a diet in which you are directed to drink a concoction of lemon juice, purified water, maple syrup and cayenne pepper for up to two weeks, contains no protein, no minerals or vitamins except C, and no fat. This type of diet is potentially dangerous and promotes starvation. Loss of copper, potassium, magnesium and other nutrients can be dangerous and lead to heart arrhythmias, impaired immunity or other medical problems.

In order to be a proper, and realistic (non-fad) diet, the diet and exercise program should, realistically, target weight loss of about one to two pounds per week. The problem with some of the intensive, calorie-restricting diets that promote weight loss of more than two to three pounds per week, is that they will promote loss of both fat and lean skeletal muscle. This is bad. In this book we have repeatedly emphasized and focus on the need to rebuild lean skeletal muscle. Severe calorie restriction will have the opposite effect. Skeletal muscle will be lost, and your overall metabolic rate will actually decrease. Then, when you go back to your old eating habits because this severe calorie restriction is not sustainable. You will gain more weight quickly and store it as fat, having lost even more skeletal muscle during this "fasting/severe calorie restriction" type of diet. The net result of Yo-Yo dieting is a body with a higher body fat percentage, which negatively affects your health and your appearance.

Another clue that a fad diet is not healthy is if it is very restrictive, and only allows you to eat a few foods or instructs you to avoid entire food groups. These diets keep you from getting all the nutrients that you need for good health. Most of these fad diets do not encourage you to eat a balanced diet that includes fruits, vegetables, whole grains, low-fat dairy products, nuts and lean proteins. Many fad diets are based on proprietary diet foods you need to purchase from the diet company.

Fad diets are also characterized by being not sustainable. In many cases these diets restrict your calories or your food options so much that you are too hungry or too bored with your food options to continue with the diet. These types of diets set you up for yo-yo dieting. After you give up on the fad diet, you quickly regain the weight you lost and often add even more.

Fad diets appeal to consumers because they are pitched in a way that sounds too good to be true. Some diets promise that you will lose tremendous amounts of weight very quickly while you continue to eat as much as you want. They may even claim that you don't have to exercise to accomplish this weight loss. They show before and after pictures, often with digital enhancements to the pictures. Testimonials often accompany the photos. They pay celebrities to endorse their plan, even when they do not follow it. No healthy diet can deliver the results claimed, but Americans literally "eat it up." Guess what. If it sounds too good to be true, it is.

Some fad diets also include appetite suppressants, with false claims about revving up your metabolism. There is very little if any science to suggest that there are safe, non-prescription pills that will either promote faster metabolism or "burn fat." These are common claims of many diet pills or food "supplements." It is amazing that the FDA allows these types of claims in health food stores with little or no scientific evidence. When you see these claims of fat burning or metabolism enhancing pills you should generally run the other way. One should also be very careful before taking any of these supplements to make certain that they do not interact in a dangerous way with any prescribed medications that you are taking.

The FDA has just recently approved a new prescription diet pill, Belviq. This is the first FDA approved diet pill in 13 years. Belviq works along with proper diet and exercise to potentially help with weight loss. It works directly on the brain to increase satiety by affecting the Serotonin 2C receptor, in a part of the brain that helps to regulate appetite. The long term risks of this drug are not fully known and like other diet pills, it may carry some risks. If you follow the rules and program of this book, you should not need this type of expensive and potentially risky, prescription drug.

In the long run, dieters that have tried, and skipped from one fad diet plan to the next will eventually get discouraged. The American Council on Exercise reports that only five percent of dieters who use these types of dietary plans manage to keep their lost weight off. On the other hand, successful dieters who adopt a more balanced, slower and sustainable weight loss plan, which embraces moderate calorie restriction with exercise, have kept off an average of sixty-six pounds for at least five years. Despite the allure, the benefits of fad diets are limited. A fad diet may only set you up for failure, decrease your metabolism and increase your risk of health problems. Since fad diets market themselves as the easiest way to lose weight, and the key to success, you may develop the feeling that you can never lose weight. This is not true.

You can achieve a healthy and sustainable weight loss by following the dietary eating guidelines in Chapter Five and by enhancing your metabolic rate by slowly building metabolically active skeletal muscle. As we have repeatedly emphasized in this book, the key is eating fewer calories than you burn (two plus two equals four). This is all that is required to lose weight. You do not have to give up entire food groups. If this does not resonate yet, re-read Chapter Five.

Fad Exercise Plans

There are almost as many fad exercise plans as fad diets. Hyped, fad exercise programs have been around for a long time. I could write a book twice as long as this entire book just listing and briefly describing more than five-hundred fad exercise programs promoted in the last decade. You could fill a large living room with one set of the videotapes, CDs, DVDs, and exercise paraphernalia from these fad exercise programs in ads, books, magazines and infomercials from the last decade. Similar to fad diets, these fad exercise plans take advantage of the weaknesses of the American consumer by promising rapid or nearly immediate results, with a money-back guarantee. Like fad diets many of these exercise programs are not realistic or sustainable over a lifetime. These programs typically are promoted with infomercials, and require the consumer to buy a dozen or more DVDs, along with a variety of exercise equipment supplements such as stretch bands, abdominal exercising equipment, or other equipment that is marked up to maximize the Visa bill when you call in to get thin in thirty days.

Like fad diets, if you could plug in the DVD and spend an hour a day, six days per week doing exactly what the fad exercise promoters teach, it will work. However, also like most fad diets, most individuals who "invest" in these DVDs and accessory equipment will end up putting them in the back of the closet within two to three months. Not sustainable.

One of the famous workout celebrities recently promoted a book to get thin in thirty days. What you should you do after the thirty days is over is not entirely clear. This book prescribes a very specific set of exercises for each day. Many of these exercises are exercises that only a super-fit athlete could possibly perform, like leaning backward balancing with one hand on a large exercise ball, and doing dumbbell exercises with the other hand while balancing on the ball. There is no way that 95% of overweight adults could even begin to do many of these prescribed exercises. However, this was a New York Times bestseller, because the woman on the cover was hot, had a great body, and was famous. This is the stereotypical fad exercise program. Americans bought it, even though it makes very little sense. Remember, a good eating and fitness program is not about fitting into a dress for a wedding next month.

One of the most extreme and successful new workout fads is P90X. This was even promoted in an article in the New York Times, describing how some younger, ex-military congressmen were trying it. This is an extreme workout from day one. It is a program that is totally unrealistic for 90% of overweight, middle aged adults. The exercise is too extreme. It starts at a high level of fitness, to take fit individuals to extreme fitness. It can work for fit and highly motivated, younger individuals. However, the goals and target audience for P90X and a dozen or so spin-off super-fitness fad-exercise programs are completely different than the target for this book.

Recently there have been a few fad programs that are starting to focus on the key elements emphasized in this book. The recent "10-Minute" workout is focusing on high intensity short duration workouts. Of course even this is flawed since it is appealing, again, to the get fixed quick mentality of Americans. The high intensity, stacking concept of stressing multiple muscle groups in one exercise is a very good concept, but 10 minutes is definitely not enough time to get a good high intensity stress to all of your muscle groups unless you do it 3-4 times per day, three days per week. That is much more disruptive and possibly less effective than the 30-40 minutes three times a week proposed in the Burn Calories approach. So, even the newer fad programs that are starting to get at the real issue of metabolic change using high intensity, short duration workouts have gone "super fad" by trying to do it in 7-10 minutes. This is just another form of hype and marketing used by almost all of these fad exercise programs. Ultimately, the large majority of both fad diets and fad exercising are proposing approaches that are un-teachable, un-learnable and not sustainable. This is why they usually fail to achieve the promised results.

In contrast to these infomercial, celebrity-backed, slick, fad-exercise programs, the Burn Calories approach allows even unfit, overweight individuals to start at a stress level that they can tolerate. With this program you can start with a low amount of weight and relatively few repetitions, with exercises that can be performed by adults who have no athletic talent. As you get more comfortable with stressing your body and breathing hard you will get stronger. This will not happen in few weeks, but over a few months. As you get stronger and more comfortable with breathing hard, and the high intensity aerobic weight lifting, you will begin to add weight and reps. When you combine this with crunches in your car, isometric fidgeting and better eating "rules," and see the results of greater strength and balance, shrinking waist size, and feeling high energy, the positive feedback will make this program sustainable. Not just for thirty days, but for your lifetime. Importantly, the program is realistic, achievable and very time efficient. Eventually, you will feel like an athlete, perhaps for the first time in your life. That is the goal.

CHAPTER SIX KEY POINTS: FAD DIETS AND EXERCISING

1) Fad diets and fad exercise programs appeal to Americans' psyche.

2) You will always see amazing "before" and "after" pictures!

3) These programs promise immediate and dramatic results in very short periods of time.

4) The programs are generally "too good to be true," and that is correct.

5) Severe calorie restriction diets can be dangerous.

6) Some diets can promote skeletal muscle loss and decrease metabolism.

7) Fad diets and fad exercising are not sustainable for most people.

8) If you don't believe Rule #6, look in the back of your closet for exercise DVDs.

❧ *Chapter Seven* ❧

Know Your Cholesterol: Do You Want to Die From a Heart Attack at Age 50 or Cancer at Age 90?

There are some very important numbers that impact your life. Maybe the most important is your age, which at some level also predicts your life expectancy. As you get older you begin to realize that all you really have is time and the health to enjoy that time. This book is about turning back the clock and trying to dissociate chronological age form biological age. In other words, we want to make you a 55 year old, chronologically, who is a 40 or 45 year old biologically.

Other important numbers in your life could be your social security number, your income, your wedding anniversary date, the amount of debt on your home, etc. There is one very important number that nearly 50% of Americans do not even know. It is the measurement of their blood or serum, cholesterol level. Even more specifically, your LDL (low density lipoprotein = bad cholesterol and your HDL (high density lipoprotein) = good cholesterol. Although the percentage of American adults who have had their

135

cholesterol checked with a blood test may now be approaching 70%, probably less than half of these adults know what their cholesterol reading is, and many of these individuals are left untreated despite unacceptably high cholesterol levels.

What if I told you that those lipid value "numbers" may be the single most important predictor or how long, and to some degree how healthily you will live your life. You need to know this number! If these numbers are very unhealthy, you will develop premature atherosclerosis and either die or be disabled by a heart attack or stroke or other consequences of this disease in your 50s or 60s for men or in your 60s-70s for women. If you can work on achieving very low cholesterol, there is good news and bad news. The good news is that you will probably not die from a heart attack or a stroke at a young age. The bad news is that you will still die, but probably from cancer at an advanced age, like 90.

Women have some protection from atherosclerosis during their pre-menopausal life due to beneficial effects of female hormones (both estrogen and progesterone) on lipids. This is mainly in the form of high HDL (good cholesterol) that protects women to some degree for 40-50 years. However, as you should know the women catch up pretty quickly after menopause when those hormone levels drop. In fact, atherosclerosis and coronary artery disease is so accelerated in women after menopause that despite the protection that women are afforded in their premenopausal years, they catch up quickly with men, such that the number one killer of women in the U.S. and other western countries is coronary heart disease and heart attacks, not breast cancer, as some may think. Heart disease kills three times more women than breast cancer. Recently the Go Red campaign has tried to educate women about this. We will talk a little more about women and their issues including heart disease in the chapter devoted to women-specific health issues in Chapter Ten.

Let's get back to cholesterol now for both men and women. Why are these lipid numbers so critical? LDL, in particular and some of the other low-density lipoproteins (e.g., VLDL) are dangerous. These lipids damage the lining of your arteries. Over many years this will cause inflammation, and the growth of atherosclerotic plaques inside your arteries supplying blood to your heart, brain, kidneys, legs, etc. Initially (in your 20s and 30s) the arteries, including the heart (coronary) arteries can compensate for the buildup of this scar tissue and fat deposits inside the artery wall by growing outward or enlarging the artery. We call this positive remodeling of the artery.

Eventually the plaques get even bigger, and begin to encroach on the lumen (opening) of the arteries. Many of the plaques develop a lipid core or fat deposit inside the plaque. This fat deposit often has a thin layer of fibrous tissue overlying it, yielding a very dangerous type of plaque called a TCFA (thin capped fibro-atheroma). We know that these are basically slow ticking time bombs that can break open like a pimple and erupt fat into the artery lumen, promoting the formation of a blood clot inside the artery and starting a heart attack or a stroke. This is very dangerous and can kill or disable you at a relatively young age. We all have friends or relatives that have had a massive, disabling or fatal strokes or heart attacks in their 30s, 40s or 50s.

When does atherosclerosis start?

Somewhat shockingly this disease process of atherosclerosis starts at a very young age especially in children and young adults eating a typical high fat and fast food diet. In the Vietnam War scientists looked at the aorta and other large arteries in eighteen-year-old soldiers who were killed in battle. At the age of eighteen, these young men had the early signs of atherosclerosis with fatty streaks of plaque buildup in their aorta and other arteries. These findings are pretty scary, and are relevant to the concept of "primary" versus "secondary" prevention of atherosclerosis. So, if you are over the age of thirty and you live in the United States or another "modern" country where McDonalds, Kentucky Fried Chicken and Taco Bell are present, and you want to know if you have atherosclerosis, the answer is YES. You have the disease.

Primary versus Secondary Atherosclerosis Prevention and Treatment

A number of medical societies and advisory groups including the prominent National Cholesterol Education Program (NCEP), have differentiated the recommendations for cholesterol lowering for primary prevention of atherosclerosis (i.e., in people who have never had any symptoms or events related to atherosclerosis) from secondary prevention (i.e., people who have had clinical events such as heart attack or stroke). The current guidelines also emphasize the target for LDL (bad) cholesterol lowering as a function of one's underlying risk of developing clinical events from atherosclerosis. For example, in the 2011 guidelines the NCEP recommendations would suggest that the target for LDL lowering would be an LDL as high as 160 mg/dl in individuals at low risk of developing a heart attack (i.e., primary prevention). The guidelines do recommend a more aggressive LDL lowering in patients who are at high risk or who have had clinical events such as a heart attack (i.e., secondary prevention). In these higher risk individuals they recommend lowering LDL to 100 mg/dl and, when possible, to as low as 70 mg/dl.

On face value these recommendations make some sense. That is, we should be more worried about individuals who have established disease or have already had a heart attack. On the other hand, this is in some ways as silly as our old approach to what was an "acceptable" cholesterol level.

We used to look at the whole U.S. population and look at the average cholesterol. If your cholesterol was within about 50-100 mg/dl of this average value we used to say, "You're fine, because your cholesterol level is normal." In this setting the word normal is a statistical term, meaning that your level of cholesterol is not dramatically different from average value in the population. The problem with this and the problem even with the more aggressive NCEP guidelines is that they are asking the wrong question. The question is not, "Is your cholesterol normal?", because it is normal in this population of adults for the men to drop dead from massive heart attacks in their 30s and 40s. The correct question is not what is normal, but what is healthy.

We are born with a cholesterol level of about 60-70 mg/dl. Animals that are mainly vegetarians and do not eat ice cream or fast food also typically have LDL cholesterol levels of 60-70 mg/dl. Giraffes and rabbits do not die from heart attacks. Do you want to be like a rabbit or giraffe with regard to stroke and heart attack risk or like the eighteen-year-old Vietnam War soldiers who were killed in battle and were found to and already have atherosclerosis in their teens?

I believe that this distinction between primary prevention and secondary prevention of atherosclerosis is an artificial distinction. It is misleading. If you are over the age of thirty, eat an American diet, and want to know if you have atherosclerosis, the answer is YES. So in fact all treatments and targets should be based upon the knowledge that everyone who eats a western diet or who has other risk factors such as high blood pressure, diabetes, obesity, sedentary lifestyle, or smoking has this disease. This concept of primary and secondary prevention does not make much sense and should be eliminated! The only thing we should focus on is—what is healthy and the prevention of atherosclerosis.

We should be asking, "What is the healthiest level of cholesterol and LDL that we can achieve?" Can we get our cholesterol to levels as low as they were when we were born, and as low as herbivores, who do eat meat or fats, and do not develop atherosclerosis? Can we raise the good cholesterol (HDL) to the highest level that we can achieve? Can we get our ratio (the ratio of total cholesterol divided by the good (HDL) cholesterol) to 3.0 or less? These should be the targets if we want to have the chance to nearly eliminate the disabling or mortal clinical events caused by atherosclerosis.

LOWERING "BAD" CHOLESTEROL (LDL)

Low-density lipoprotein, or LDL, is the evil or bad cholesterol. We do need LDL and cholesterol in the body to make hormones, to maintain the cell membranes and for other important functions. However, at high levels LDL does a number of bad things when it is in your blood and exposed to your blood vessel wall. High levels of LDL can damage the function of the endothelium, which are the important lining cells on the inside of your arteries. LDL can get attached to the blood vessel wall and incorporated into the inner layer of an artery, inciting inflammation. It can attract white blood cells into the blood vessel wall that release growth factors to stimulate the growth of atherosclerotic plaque buildup inside the artery. The sharp edged cholesterol crystals in the LDL may actually be able to cause physical rupture of the plaque and trigger a heart attack.

I have already told you my bias. The correct LDL is the lowest that we can reasonably achieve, even if this requires some modest drug intervention. Scientists have not yet found point of LDL lowering that causes adverse effects, and does not lower cardiovascular risk. A target LDL of 60-70 mg/dl, sustained for a lifetime will nearly eliminate the risk of having a major heart attack. There are very few Americans or any other adult humans who will achieve this low level of LDL without excellent genetics, and/or incredible diets and regular vigorous exercise. Even with a very good diet and exercise this low level of LDL may be difficult to achieve without some help from medication.

Unfortunately, most individuals have already had the normal boundaries of their LDL level set, in large part, by their heredity. The genetics of LDL metabolism is highly influenced by the DNA that you inherited from your parents. This is the main reason that a strong family history of premature coronary heart disease and heart attacks is a pretty potent risk factor for having one yourself. If your mother or father or uncle or aunt had heart a heart attack or bypass surgery in their 40s or 50s, you absolutely need to know your cholesterol and your LDL levels. If you have this type of family history, it is most often related to the genetics of your family's cholesterol metabolism. This does not necessarily mean that you have a high cholesterol and LDL. It also does not mean that you are doomed to repeat the history of your parent(s) who suffered from a heart attack or cardiac death at a young age. It does mean that the set-point, or range for your LDL is likely to be higher than someone without this family history. It may mean, in some cases that the genetics of your cholesterol handling is so bad, that it may not be possible to get your LDL to a healthy level with even the greatest diet and fanatic exercise. It may mean that you will need to make lifestyle interventions and take medication to achieve a truly healthy level of LDL. There are some great tips about a novel way to use statins the highly potent drug for LDL lowering in the later part of this chapter.

Let's outline the key ways that we can get you to the target of healthy LDL in the 70 mg/dl range, even if you have bad genetics. The first key intervention is typically referred to as lifestyle changes. This basically means better eating and more physical exercise. Let's focus briefly on the eating.

There is no question that cholesterol and LDL are closely linked to your diet. There are thousands of articles and hundreds of books that you can refer to guide you to a "heart healthy" diet. This book is not going to have a hundred pages about this type of diet, since almost everyone reading this book can already recite the kinds of foods that will raise your cholesterol. Basically, fatty foods, fried foods and foods that have very high intrinsic cholesterol content like liver, spleen, kidney, egg yolks and brain will raise your LDL. Luckily, most people do not really like or eat the liver and brain. However, the fast-food, fatty diets which have massive caloric content also typically have a very high cholesterol content. Fast food should be avoided or eliminated from your diet.

Egg yolks also have a lot of cholesterol and should be eaten in moderation. If you like eggs it is best to eat egg whites or egg beaters, etc. One great trick to cut the cholesterol content in eggs (like omelets) to 1/2 to 1/3 of usual is to make your scrambled eggs or omelets with a combination of one egg yolk for every 3-4 egg whites. In this way the eggs still look yellow and taste amazingly identical to eggs with a full complement of yolks. This is just another great little pearl. This will allow you to eat eggs with their great protein content and yet avoid eating high intake of cholesterol.

The best diet to nearly eliminate cholesterol intake is a vegetarian diet. There are very few vegetable sources of cholesterol, so if one eats vegetarian and eliminates egg yolks, you can achieve a nearly cholesterol free diet. As I tell my patients, the closer you can get to eating like a rabbit the better. There is a strong correlation between cholesterol lowering diets and diets that will help with your weight loss. So, the double bonus for those who can nearly eliminate fried foods, fatty foods and meat from their diet is achieving both low cholesterol and weight loss.

Unfortunately, for some people with very bad genetics, one can still have a high LDL even when you don't eat any foods that contain cholesterol. This ties in to some of the critical pearls about lowering LDL in this chapter. The cholesterol in your blood does not only come from cholesterol that is ingested. Cholesterol is synthesized inside your body. The liver is the main site for cholesterol production. This is why you can eat very little cholesterol or fat and still have an elevated cholesterol and LDL.

This is the part that is genetic, so if you don't like it, yell at your parents!

Medication to Lower the Bad (LDL) Cholesterol

So, if diet and exercise have not allowed you to achieve the very healthy target of an LDL in the range of 70-80 mg/dl, it is time to think about medication to achieve this aggressive target. There are a number of medications that have been proven to do this, including the drugs called statins, as well as cholesterol binding agents and some other relatively weak medicines. I like to focus on the statins because they are relatively safe, easy to take and highly effective in lowering LDL and total cholesterol. This class of drugs also has, by far, the most compelling scientific studies showing that lowering LDL with these agents can prevent heart attacks and stroke and will prolong life. This is a very important class of drug.

The number one problem with taking statins (Lipitor, Zocor, Crestor, Mevacor, Lescol, etc.) for many patients is that it often causes quite severe muscle aching. We call this myalgia (pain in the muscles). The exact cause of this is not well understood, but it clearly is a common side effect of this drug when taken on a daily basis. It is by far the number one reason that many patients and their doctors give up and stop taking this important class of medicine. Taking high doses of these drugs on a daily basis may also rarely cause liver damage. This needs to be monitored with blood tests.

Here is the bad news and good news, and perhaps the most life-saving tip in this book. Almost all adults need to take statins in order to get to life saving, very low levels of LDL in their blood, but these drugs DO NOT need to be taken every day. The drug companies, who want to sell as much of these drugs as possible do not want you to know that taking these medications just 2-3 times per week is adequate to dramatically reduce your cholesterol (more on this in a minute). The benefits to taking the medication only 2-3 times per week are: 1) The drug is now less than half the price. Your doctor can still prescribe it on an everyday schedule. In this way you need fewer refills if you are taking it every second or third day. 2) This every second or third day dosing will dramatically reduce, but not completely eliminate, the side effects of muscle pain (myalgia) and liver damage (to be explained in next paragraph). 3) Your LDL and total cholesterol will drop by 30-40%, or more, especially when combined with a good diet and a good (Burn Calories) exercise program that stresses skeletal muscle.

So why take the statin only every 3rd day? Here is the secret that your doctor and the drug companies have not told you or do not think about. It is not the statin medication per se that lowers your total cholesterol and your LDL. It is your liver. Although the drug itself causes the side effects (like myalgia) the drug only acts as a messenger, of sorts, to give the liver the message to remove cholesterol from your blood and thereby lower your cholesterol. The drug, itself, in the bloodstream does not lower the cholesterol. How does this work?

The statin drug goes into the liver and blocks the liver's ability to make cholesterol by blocking a critical enzyme in the liver cell that is the rate-limiting step in the liver cell's quest to make cholesterol (the enzyme that is blocked by statins is called HMG CoA-Reductase in case you wanted to impress your friends). Cholesterol is needed in the body and in the liver to be put into cell membranes, make hormones, etc. When the statin is in the liver cell it cannot make enough cholesterol in the liver cell. The liver now feels deprived of cholesterol since its own internal machinery has been disabled. So, the liver decides to go get cholesterol and LDL out of the blood. When deprived of internally produced cholesterol, the liver turns on the machinery to make LDL receptors and put these receptors (proteins) on its own cell membrane. The liver cell (hepatocyte) turns on its messenger RNA that gives the instructions to make LDL receptors. The liver cell starts making a lot of these receptors and they migrate to the cell membrane of the liver cell. These new LDL receptors then filter the blood, literally sucking LDL particles out of the passing blood. This is how the statins have their potent effect in reducing the cholesterol and LDL in your blood.

Once you have made these protein receptors they last for at least 30 days on the liver cell surface. Here is the key point. You do not need to tell the liver to make these new receptors every day. If you take the statin even every 3rd or 4th day, you will keep up a great concentration of LDL receptors on the liver cells, and keep sucking the LDL out of your blood and away from harming your blood vessels. This is a great pearl for nearly all adults. My own LDL had drifted up over many years from 80 to 85 then eventually to 98. I realized that although this was still relatively low and well below the "primary prevention" guidelines, it was still high enough to promote atherosclerosis and cause a heart attack in my 60s or 70s. If that is the case one might naturally ask the question, "Why not lower the LDL to a very low level and lower the risk?" So, I started taking atorvastatin (Lipitor) at a very low dose of only 10 mg every 3rd day. Even though I admittedly do not follow a great diet (I do like cheeseburgers), when this low dose of satin was combined high-intensity, short-duration exercise twice a week, my LDL dropped from 98 to 52 in 2 years! This is a very low LDL that was achieved with high intensity weight lifting twice a week, a reasonable but not restrictive diet, and most importantly, with low dose statin taken every 3rd day. You need to check your cholesterol and get to these targets (LDL 70) if you want to help to prevent and even possibly reverse atherosclerosis.

RAISING "GOOD" CHOLESTEROL (HDL)

High-density lipoprotein, or HDL, is the good cholesterol. Unlike LDL, which is directly correlated with increasing your risk of atherosclerosis, heart attack and stroke, the HDL has an inverse correlation. This means that the higher your HDL, the lower your risk of developing a heart attack or cardiac death. In fact, a high HDL is more protective unit for unit than LDL is harmful. For every 10 mg/dl the HDL is actually three times more protective than the LDL is harmful. So, you are actually much more protected with a high HDL than you are with a low LDL.

Men are particularly at risk here since it appears that testosterone may lower HDL. In contrast women have a great benefit from female hormones of estrogen and progesterone, which appear to significantly increase HDL in women, at least until they reach the menopause. Not too surprisingly, once women lose the high levels of these hormones, their lipids begin to look more like men's' and their risk of heart attack and stroke rises dramatically.

One of the great challenges, however, is making any manipulations in lifestyle or with drugs that will beneficially effect and raise your HDL. The most powerful way to raise one's HDL, for both men and women is to exercise very vigorously. Aerobic exercise will raise the HDL. Importantly, it appears that weight training may be even more effective in raising the HDL. This is one reason that the high intensity skeletal muscle stress from the Burn Calories workout pays even bigger dividends, by lowering LDL and raising HDL.

How about medications to raise HDL? There are a number of medications that are known to raise the HDL. These drugs include niacin/nicotinic acid, fish oils, gemfibrizol and a few others.

Historically, the most commonly used drug has been nicotinic acid. One of the more popular formulations of this drug is call Niaspan. It is a little longer-acting and has fewer side effects of flushing than niacin. Up until recently it was assumed that the HDL raising effect of Niaspan would significantly decrease the risk of heart attack, stroke and cardiac death. However, in one of the largest, and very recent studies in which Niaspan was compared to placebo (sugar pills), the Niaspan did raise the HDL, as expected, but it had no effect on cardiac death or heart attacks.

These new data are somewhat shocking to many of us who felt that raising HDL would be at least as potent, if not more powerful than lowering LDL as a means to prevent heart attacks and strokes. However, this newer negative study is the second recent major study to suggest that using medication to raise HDL may not confer risk reduction benefit. The other recent study looked at a potentially exciting new class of drugs that can dramatically increase the HDL. The drug tested in this case was called Torcetribid. In this study, once again, the patients taking the drug had a major increase in their HDL level, but they actually had a slightly higher risk of cardiovascular events. This was surprising to many scientists who have studied the effects of HDL on lowering cardiac risk. This drug will, of course, never get FDA approved. In summary, these two large studies, sadly, cast a shadow over the entire concept of drug manipulations to lower HDL in order to lower cardiovascular risk.

It appears that the best we can do for now is to make lifestyle manipulations including vigorous exercise, with a focus on weight training. This will predictably help to raise HDL, without medication. One other good news is that alcohol will also raise HDL and may confer reduced cardiac risk. As far as we can tell, it does not matter what form the alcohol is in (i.e., vodka, red wine, white wine, beer, etc.). It appears to be the alcohol itself that modestly raises HDL and lowers cardiac risk. So drink up, but remember rule 10 in the eating rules!

A New concept: "Non-HDL Cholesterol"?

Primary care physicians and cardiologists have finally begun to focus on primary and secondary prevention of cardiovascular events by treating high cholesterol and high LDL. Based upon a wealth of scientific information, this makes great sense. As discussed above, there are challenges in raising the good cholesterol and uncertainty about the value of trying to raise the good cholesterol (HDL) with medications.

More recently, lipid experts have focused on another part of the lipid profile called Non-HDL cholesterol. What is this? This is all of the cholesterol that is found in other lipoprotein molecules that are not LDL or HDL. These molecules include VLDL (very low density lipoprotein), IDL (intermediate density lipoprotein) and some other even rarer forms of cholesterol carrying molecules. In the last 10 years we have recognized that these other non-HDL cholesterol carrying molecules, like LDL, can promote atherosclerosis. Recent studies have demonstrated that the value of non-HDL cholesterol is actually a better long-term predictor of risk of heart attack and stroke than the more traditional LDL cholesterol value.

A Critical Number! What is Your Ratio?

Last but not least, one of the most critical predictors of atherosclerosis risk is a ratio of the total cholesterol divided by the good cholesterol (HDL). If you get a lipid profile blood test drawn by your doctor this "ratio" will almost always be a part of the report. What is "healthy?" Well, ideally the ratio of total cholesterol divided by the HDL should be 3.0. With a good diet, exercise, a statin, and maybe a little alcohol chaser this ratio can be achieved by most people. This is usually pretty easy for women, who are blessed with relatively high HDLs, especially prior to menopause.

So, if you want to live to 90, know your cholesterol and your "ratio." If these are not at the targets described in this chapter, make it a priority to get to these targets, by diet and exercise. If diet and exercise are not enough due to your genetics, which is the case for most people, you may need a statin! Take it 2-3 times per week and you can afford it, tolerate it and hit these life-saving targets for cholesterol.

CHAPTER SEVEN KEY POINTS: CHOLESTEROL AND LIPIDS

1) Know your number! What is your total cholesterol, LDL, HDL and ratio?

2) These numbers predict your life expectancy and risk of heart attack & stroke!

3) Dietary and lifestyle changes are critical to get to a healthy level of cholesterol.

4) Atherosclerosis (hardening of arteries) begins in childhood.

5) If you are over the age of 40 and have not been perfect, you have this disease!

6) Younger women are protected from atherosclerosis, but catch up quickly after menopause.

7) LDL is the bad cholesterol and needs to be as low as possible.

8) Current targets for primary prevention are too high (LDL should be 70-80).

9) Most adults will need medication (statin) to get to very low LDL levels.

10) Statins taken only 2-3 times per week yields great results; less side effects.

11) Natural ways to raise HDL (good cholesterol) are important and include exercise (weight lifting) and modest alcohol. Drugs may not work.

❧ *Chapter Eight* ❧

TEACH YOUR CHILDREN WELL: HOW TO STOP THE OBESITY EPIDEMIC

CHILDREN ARE ONE THIRD OF OUR POPULATION, AND ALL OF OUR FUTURE.

(Select Panel for the Promotion of Child Health, 1981)

Children are our future. The battle against the obesity epidemic in the United States, and in other modern countries has to start with our children. Childhood obesity has soared to record levels. We are seeing children in their early teens with morbid obesity and even type 2 diabetes. We must do a better job at multiple levels in caring for and educating our children. We must be role models for them in demonstrating, promoting and teaching healthy lifestyle and eating habits. We must follow and teach the "10 Rules" of eating to our children. It would be great to do a family Burn Calories workout together 2-3 times per week. This chapter will focus on just how dangerous and life altering it will be if we let our children eat too much, be physically inactive and become overweight. If we care about our children's health and the "health" of the citizens of our country going forward we must attack the problem by teaching our children well. Unfortunately, many parents in our society force, encourage, or allow their children to massively overeat and develop maladaptive eating behaviors. The parents need to take more responsibility and teach their children about proper eating rules, and nutrition. Only in this way will we ever begin to really attack the root cause of the obesity epidemic in America.

Childhood Obesity in America: The Problem

Never in the history of the U.S. has there been a bigger problem with childhood obesity. More than 50% of children under the age of twelve are overweight or obese. The causes of this are complex and multifactorial. Our children are less active today than the children of the prior generation. TV, videogames, iPads, online chatting, etc. have replaced the outside activities that I grew up with as a child, such as whiffle ball, basketball, playing soldiers or war games running around the neighborhood, riding bicycles, swimming, walking to a friend's house. Now it is all done online and in cars. Kids watch and average of fourteen hours a week of television. The average ten- to fifteen-year-old spends another 12-20 hours a week on social (computer networks) or chatting on their cell phones. This has eroded a lot of interpersonal social interactions of the real world, and has promoted inactivity, lack of physical exercise and obesity. When we layer the massive caloric loads of today's fast foods on top of this inactive lifestyle and inadequate teaching of the fundamental rules of eating (re-read Chapter Five), we get obese children and an obese nation, in crisis.

Physical activity and exercise as a key life activity for children is a critical concept. Strenuous physical activity has many benefits for children. Not only does it promote being thin and fit, it also will enhance bone growth. This is particularly important for girls so that they can reduce the likelihood of osteoporosis in their later adult years. The promotion of physical activity for children is now being more actively promoted. I applaud the NFL and others for starting programs such as "Play 60." This means that all children should engage in at least 60 minutes of active physical activities, exercise or sports every day. This is a very important goal. The new rule should be, "No TV or videogames until you have had your "Play 60" fix.

Obesity in childhood carries with it a number of major negative health consequences. Childhood obesity is linked to high blood pressure and high cholesterol, increased risk of type 2 diabetes, breathing problems including sleep apnea and asthma, joint and musculosketal problems, gallstones and acid reflux (heartburn), as well as a greater risk of social and psychological problems, including discrimination and low self-esteem which can carry forward into adulthood. Obesity is not "OK."

Fat Begets Fat

It is not well known to most parents but the number of fat cells that we ultimately have as an adult is not preset at birth, but is determined in large part, by how much we eat (or overeat) and our thinness, or obesity status as a child. Fat cells (adipocytes) are capable of dividing and growing in numbers during childhood. If we eat well and exercise and if we are thin as children, we will have a relatively smaller number of fat cells. If we overeat and do all the wrong things and we are obese as children, we may have 2-3 fold the number of fat cells at age twelve than our thinner twelve-year-old next-door neighbor. Why is the number of fat cells that we have at age twelve important? Because the number of fat cells that you will have for the rest of your life is pretty well fixed at about age twelve to thirteen. Fat cells will divide up to that time and then we stop making new fat cells. Short of liposuction, or other surgical procedure to mechanically remove these fat cells, we will be stuck with these extra billions of fat cells for the rest of our lives.

This, among other reasons, is why fat children become fat adults. It is why attacking the obesity epidemic by teaching our children well is so critical. The mass of fat cells that you have helps to regulate your hunger and satiety patterns for the rest of your life. Fat, as an organ system, sends out hormonal messages,

159

including the important hormone known as leptin. These hormones play an important role in the regulation of hunger and satiety. Unfortunately, if you have 3 times more fat cells you may have three times the appetite. This is one of the reasons that adults who were overweight as children often to have a tough time with dieting and maintaining a healthy weight.

FOCUSING ON RULES OF EATING FOR OUR CHILDREN

Hopefully the Rules of Eating as outlined in Chapter Five are still fresh in your mind. These key rules are as critical for our children as they are for us, as adults. If fact, several of the rules are really based upon the distorted eating rules that were taught and imposed upon many of us in the 1950s, 1960s and 1970s (and even now) growing up. How many of us, as children, were told to clear everything on your plate? "You should not waste food!" "There are children starving in China (or India)!" Did Mom or Dad ever really intend to take the leftover food, place it in a box and FedEx it to children in New Delhi? Of course not. But, it made us feel guilty and imposed a set of eating behaviors to eat everything on our plate, and not to waste food. We were taught that it was better to stuff ourselves way past full and clean our plate rather than follow Rule #2, i.e., "When you are full, you are done!"

Cleaning off all of the food on your plate was praised. Asking for seconds was praised because it made Mom feel like she was a good cook. If somehow you did not eat any portion of your meal Mom would often take it as a personal insult to her cooking, so the children were guilted into eating anything and everything on your plate, and more than you wanted or needed to eat. It did not matter that the kids were eating way beyond their satiety, and with an extra 2,000 calories per day that they did not want or need. It was more important that they ate a lot of food, cleared their plate, praised Mom's cooking and did not waste food. So what if they were stimulating the growth a few billion extra fat cells that would end up torturing them for the rest of their adult life, as they jumped from fad diet to fad diet, trying to erase the damage from a childhood "filled" with praise and rewards for overeating.

This deviant and maladaptive eating behavior was often further reinforced by our parents telling us that there was a reward for eating past full, and stuffing our face with 100's or even 1,000's of extra calories. Yes, if we cleared our plate we could have desert! Wow, if we eat 500 calories more than we can stand the reward is a 500-calorie piece of Mom's fresh chocolate cake. This is how we get Rule #3: "Dessert is NOT a reward for breaking Rule #2." This type of eating messaging is another contributor to the creation of obese children, and adults who will fight with their extra weight their whole lives. Let's stop the maladaptive teaching and start teaching eating rules (Chapter Five) that make sense and will allow the next generation to be thin and fit!

Fast Foods and Obesity in Childhood

There is little question that to explosion of fast food chains (McDonald's, Burger King, Wendy's, Taco Bell, Jack in The Box, Kentucky Fried Chicken, Arby's, etc. etc.) has had a huge impact upon the skyrocketing rates of childhood obesity. These are quick, easy, convenient, and inexpensive, and the kids like it. So what's the big deal? Parents find it much easier to pick up a take-out pepperoni pizza or a bucket of the Colonel's delicious finger licking good grease-laden drumsticks, rather than cook a healthy meal at home. These are cheap calories. You can fill the kid's up with very little money. Fast food is cheap food. There are more calories per dollar in fast food than in healthy food either at home or at a better restaurant. It's a little like buying high-octane gasoline for $0.50/gallon. Seems great until you realize what the additives in this cheap gas are doing to our children's' engines.

The ready availability of densely caloric and inexpensive fast food is certainly one of the key drivers in the childhood obesity epidemic. Of course, as these "children" grow up into adults, and have been engrained in the fast food culture and they continue these eating habits. As they age, and become sedentary, with a decreased metabolic rate, this explodes obese children into morbidly obese and diabetic adults. Sadly, we (America) are now exporting this "fast food culture" overseas to countries like China and Japan. As a coronary/heart stent developer this is good for my business (I call it growing crops for in-the-future heart stents), but it is bad for the health of these populations. I would much rather see us export healthy habits, culture and businesses overseas.

So, for all of us parents, it is time to resist the temptation to take the easy fast food path. Ultimately, parents have the greatest opportunity to alter the frightening course and projections of adult obesity. If we teach great lifetime eating and exercising habits to our children, and act as role models, we can stop this epidemic.

CHAPTER EIGHT KEY POINTS: TEACH YOUR CHILDREN WELL

1) Remember, the # of fat cells grow until age 12; Fat children become fat adults!!

2) Follow the rules of eating with your children (Be a role model)!

3) Limit sedentary activities like TV and videogames.

4) Encourage an active lifestyle and sports. Get them outside! "Play 60."

5) Once the kids are teenagers get them lifting weights; start the habit.

6) Remember fat cells grow until age 12; fat children become fat adults!!

7) Make sure you get your children's blood pressure and lipids measured and treated if necessary.

❧ *Chapter Nine* ❧

For Men Only: Grow Hair While you Sleep, Nature's Viagra, and Other Tips

Staying Young for Men

Let's face it. None of us are getting any younger. Every day, every year, the effects of aging begin to creep up and affect us, in our looks, our weight, our energy, our sexual interest and performance, etc. Most men are less obsessed or concerned about this aging than are women, until one day we wake up, look in the mirror and say, "Who is that?" Worse yet is that revelation at the 20th high school reunion when either no one recognizes you because you have gained so much weight, lost so much hair, and just do not look anything like your high school graduation picture anymore.

Married men are generally even less concerned as they often see their wives also aging, gaining weight and say, "What the hell, I guess this is just what happens as you get older." This book and this chapter is devoted to the concept that although the aging process cannot be stopped, it can be slowed down. What are the key factors that make us look and/or feel old? The key factors are

165

our looks (weight, skin, loss and/or graying of hair, posture) our fitness and youthful drives including overall energy, stamina and, importantly, our sexual drive and potency.

In this chapter, focused on men, we are going to examine some of the key factors that either make us look or feel older, and some of the remarkably simple tips, or tricks that men can do to stay looking and feeling and acting younger. The assumption is that this is something that you want to do. That is why you bought this book and that is why you are reading it. Read on and you will get some pretty potent ways to slow down your "aging process."

BASIC WEIGHT LOSS, EATING, AND FITNESS RULES

This is just to remind you about the key elements of the book related to losing weight, and changing your metabolism by creating metabolically active and strong skeletal muscle. One of the key ways to look and feel young is to get thin, fit, and strong. This requires high intensity skeletal muscle stress and following the 10 basic rules of eating, as has been described and taught in depth in the prior chapters. Imagine if you showed up at your 20th high school reunion at your high school graduation weight, but with more muscle definition and with a six-pack. The girls/women at the reunion would be talking about you to their husbands all night. Think how many fights you could start on their drive home. "Why can't you take care of yourself...? Did you see Bob...? He looks amazing! "It goes without saying that our basic looks and energy will be highly connected to your weight and fitness. We are not going to dwell on this anymore in this chapter.

YOUR HAIR

The majority of men will face issues related to hair loss or thinning, in their lifetime. In males past their early 20s, the incidence of balding is roughly equivalent to chronological age. Thus, by age 50, roughly half of men experience male pattern baldness (also known as androgenic alopecia). Even men who are not genetically predisposed to male pattern baldness are likely to have a slow but still apparent thinning of their hair as they age. For better or worse, for most men, losing one's hair does make you look older.

If you don't care, or you like the way you look with little or no hair, or with a shaved head (Telly Savalas look) then don't worry about it. Many men are very handsome with a receding hairline. Maybe your wife or girlfriend thinks that you look distinguished, and it does not bother you at all. If that is you, skip this section. Maybe you still want to hear about tips for better sexual function, etc. so don't skip this chapter entirely.

Let's talk about hair loss and what are your options to prevent or reverse this, assuming that you do care (like most men). Male pattern baldness is very common and is characterized by loss of frontal hair and the hair on the back of your head (occiput or crown). If you want to blame someone for this, blame your mother. This is an X-linked genetic trait. This means that it was transmitted to you on the X chromosome that you got from your mother. So if you are young and you want to know if you are predisposed to have classical male pattern baldness, look at your grandfather on your mother's side (maternal grandfather) and look at your great grandfather (your mother's, mother's father) on your mother's side. If they are both bald you may want to read further about stopping hair loss, and start on a program of prevention at a relatively young age. Once you have lost your hair it will much harder to get it back.

Here is the good news. There are some scientifically validated medical options to prevent or even reverse hair loss. Men produce testosterone, primarily from the testes. This is an important hormone for male sexual characteristics, sex drive and function (more on this later). Unfortunately, the body produces a relatively toxic byproduct of testosterone called dihydro-testosterone (DHT). DHT has three major effects for men. First it stimulates the prostate gland to grow, is a contributor to prostate enlargement and probably to prostate cancer as we get older. Next, it can contribute to adult acne. Finally, it is the main (toxic) chemical responsible for damaging the hair follicle, via the androgenic receptors, in men who have the genetic susceptibility for male pattern baldness.

The increased understanding of the role of dihydrotestosterone (DHT) in male pattern baldness has led to targeted intervention to prevent this hormone from acting on scalp androgen receptors. Back in the 1980s Merck developed a drug called finasteride. The trade name for this drug is Proscar. This drug was developed and tested to help to shrink the prostate gland by blocking the conversion of testosterone to dihydrotestosterone (DHT). It worked! The drug was approved by the FDA in 1997 for the treatment of men who suffered from urinary retention due to benign prostatic hypertrophy (BPH, prostate enlargement). Recent studies have also suggested that this drug taken over many years may significantly reduce the risk of developing prostate cancer.

In the trials of this drug to treat this common prostate problem (BPH), many men who were participating in the trial made an interesting observation that was reported to Merck. They told Merck that they realized that after a few months of taking this drug that their hair was getting thicker, and that they were re-growing hair. It was this somewhat unexpected observation that ultimately led to Merck to do a clinical trial of finasteride to see if it could prevent hair loss. Even at the very low dose (1 mg/day) used in this trial, it did reduce hair loss and in some cases allow

169

hair to regrow. This drug was approved by the FDA with the indication to treat men with male pattern baldness. The dose approved to treat hair loss (1 mg/day; trade name - Propecia) is much lower than the 5 mg/day used of prostate enlargement (trade name - Proscar).

This drug really does work, and has virtually no side effects. If this drug is so good, why have so few men heard about this and why are so few taking it? First of all, the drug, Propecia, took a long time to get FDA approval for the indication of hair loss. Because of the delays in getting the drug FDA approved, the drug (finasteride) went generic pretty close to the time of the approval of Propecia. Since it was generic and, anecdotally, the 1 mg pill was less effective than the 5 mg dose, Merck never really promoted or marketed this drug for hair loss. Finally, the drug is still a prescription drug. Therefore, unless you bring this issue up with your physician, you will not be able to get the drug.

For completeness, I should mention that Dutasteride (Avodart) is very similar to finasteride (same class of medication) and also inhibits the production of DHT. However, this drug has not been as studied, or approved at any dose for the treatment of male pattern baldness.

I have personally take Proscar (5 mg/day) for nearly fifteen years with no side effects. I am biased to believe that the 5 mg dose (dose intended to treat prostate enlargement) may be a more potent dose than the 1 mg dose to prevent hair loss. I have to acknowledge that there is no scientific study behind a recommendation for 5 mg/day rather than the approved dosing of 1 mg/day. However, intuitively, the more completely you block the enzyme that helps to convert testosterone to dihydrotestosterone (DHT), perhaps the greater the protection of the hair follicle. This drug does work and will virtually halt hair loss for most men. In many cases you will appreciate that you are actually growing a lot of new hair in the border zone areas in which your hair had thinned over the years. This truly can grow hair while you sleep.

I should mention some other options to deal with male pattern baldness. The first in the topical application of the drug, minoxidil. The trade name for this medication is Rogaine. It is interesting that Rogaine has been widely marketed even though it is 1) relatively expensive, 2) only really helps some on the crown area for reducing hair loss for most men, and 3) only works in about two-thirds of men. So, this is an option. It can also be combined with finasterdide to reduce or eliminate hair loss.

Other marketed but quite unproven hair loss remedies include the herbal treatment saw palmetto, L-arginine, L-lysine, topical caffeine, phytosterols, laser light and perhaps a dozen more herbal and "home grown" and untested medical treatments. If any of them really worked almost all balding men would be using it. There has been a lot of research in the last five to ten years looking at gene therapy or even stem cell therapies to regrow hair. As of today these remain speculative, and only investigational.

Finally, for those men who either have more advanced hair loss and/or are willing to pay a lot more money and deal the discomforts of surgery, hair transplantation surgery really does work. In this procedure a physician takes hair grafts from the back of the scalp to harvest hair follicles that are genetically resistant to the toxicity of DHT. If one takes these hair follicles and transplants them to the temple or crown thinning areas, these grafts can live for your whole life and grow hair in an area on your scalp where you would not otherwise be able to grow hair. This really does work. Here are the caveats: 1) you need a really good and highly experienced surgeon to get the best results, 2) you need to get "micro grafts" (1-3 hairs moved per graft) to get a good cosmetic result without those old style plugs, that look very artificial, 3) there is a limit to how much can be transplanted, and it may take 2-3 procedures to get a very good cosmetic result for most men, 4) it is somewhat painful and takes 6-8 months after the surgery to "grow in," and finally, 5) it is expensive. So, this does work, but it is not for everyone.

A few words about gray hair. There is no doubt that graying of hair is viewed as a marker of aging. There is, of course, a pretty close correlation between age and the amount of gray hair that one has. Some men, however, may begin to be gray even in their 20s while for others, it may not really show up until nearly 60. Gray hair is caused by the reduction in the production of pigment, or melanin from the cells in the base of the hair follicle. The melanocyte cells that make pigment, for reasons that are not entirely clear, appear to fatigue and/or disappear as one ages, thus reducing the colored pigment produced with the hair in the hair follicle. There may some a condition or toxins that may accelerate this. Unfortunately, there are few, if any, medical treatments to prevent it. There is evidence that the drugs that block DHT, such as finasteride, may have some modest effect in slowing the aging process by protecting the hair follicle from the toxicity of DHT, but this is a pretty weak effect compared the effects on preventing hair loss. Graying can be associated with low vitamin B12 or thyroid hormone levels but in most cases it is just natural aging.

Some men look great with gray hair (e.g., look at Richard Gere, the actor), and have no issues with it. Even if you don't like it and think it is making you look old, the only real option to get rid of your gray hair is to shave it off or to dye it. Unlike many women, most men, will accept their gray hair, and just accept looking distinguished and "wise." Women who color their hair are cool but men look colored. Most men will not want to deal with the hassles as well as the potential embarrassment that they dye their hair. In the end, men should do whatever feels right to them.

YOUR SKIN

Just like graying of hair, skin aging is a big deal for women, who often feel that they are expected to have skin that looks like a twenty-one-year-old model. Women generally work much harder on lines and wrinkles. Most men usually do not think very much or care very much about their skin. For men it is often OK to have that aged and mature look. However, when you get huge bags under your eyes, deep wrinkles on your brow, sagging skin over your eyelids and deep lines running deeply in your nasolabial folds (those lines between your nose and the outer corners of your lips) it definitely makes you look older. If that is not important to you, skip this section. If, on the other hand you want to look 40 when you are 55 or 60, there are a number of things that men can do to reduce aging effects, and/or mask or even surgically try to reverse these age-related effects on skin.

We will start this section with the least invasive and least expensive and finish with the most invasive and most expensive. Unfortunately, there is some correlation between the amount of physical and financial pain and the effectiveness, as will be outlined below.

The cheapest and easiest way to have younger skin is to avoid things that damage and age the skin. The two critical factors here are sun and smoking. If you do not spend time in the sun and do not smoke, you will really decrease the rate of skin aging. If you do smoke, quit. If you are in the sun a lot, use SPF 30 or greater sunscreen on your face and wear a hat. Now those are the relatively simple and really inexpensive ways to protect and anti-age your skin.

What about skin creams and moisturizers? I know what most men think. This is for girls! For better or worse the cosmetic industry is now focusing more and more on skin health for men. There are some good products on the market including face scrubs (exfoliating agents) and creams that may have some modest effects on improving the health of your skin. There is a huge range and array of skin care lotions, creams and serums for men (and women). There may some small correlation between cost and efficacy, but by and large these differences are small, and there is no real science demonstrating that the $25 moisturizer is superior to the $100 bottle.

It is expensive and a little painful, but it works! I am talking about Botox. This is botulinum toxin. This is a neurotoxin that essentially paralyzes some of the small muscles in your face and reduces the effects of those muscles in causing wrinkles. This is particularly effective in the wrinkles of the forehead that many men get. It also can help with other small wrinkles, like at the corners of the eyes (crow's feet), etc. This involves injections into the skin by a trained physician. It is a prescription treatment. Although there is a little pain with the injections, the main pain is to your wallet. This will cost about $300-$1,000 per treatment, depending on how much is injected and where you live (LA probably more expensive than Des Moines). To be effective, the treatments need to be given once every 3-4 months initially. After a few years the intervals may expand out to only once every 5-6 months. This is not for everyone. However, it is one of the most effective ways, short of plastic surgery, to reduce the effects of aging on your skin.

Your Other Most Important Organ

Even if you skipped the last two sections because you are macho, Sean Connery or Lee Marvin type and don't give a c—p about the color of your hair, how much hair you have or how many wrinkles you have, most men care about their very special dual purpose organ and its health and function. If you don't care about this, then maybe you will be interested in the women's chapter. Only kidding.

Erectile dysfunction is a common medical problem, which increases with each decade of a man's age particularly after age 50.

Erectile dysfunction, commonly referred to as ED, is the inability to achieve and sustain an erection suitable for sexual intercourse. This condition is not necessarily considered normal at any age and is different from other problems that interfere with sexual intercourse, such as lack of sexual desire and problems with ejaculation and orgasm. It is a frequent problem in men who are smokers, diabetic, sedentary or who drink too much alcohol.

According to the National Institutes of Health, approximately 15% and 25% of 65-year-old men experience ED on a long-term basis. The National Institutes of Health studies have suggested that the incidence of some form of ED may be as high as 40% in men over the age of 40. In general, the incidence of ED is four times higher in men in their 60s than in men in their 40s. Thus, there is a reason that we are inundated with TV ads showing the loving couple in some romantic situation, and asks whether you (the man) will be ready when that right time comes. If you are lucky that time will come more than once every 2-3 months, unlike some marriages which will not be specifically named in this book.

Unlike true, physiologic and recurrent ED (essentially incapable of achieving an erection), the majority of men at some point in their life will be troubled occasional failure to achieve an erection. This can occur for a variety of reasons, such as from drinking too much alcohol, stress/anxiety, severe fatigue, etc.

Failure to achieve an erection less than 20% of the time is not unusual and treatment is rarely needed. Failure to achieve an erection more than 50% of the time, however, generally indicates there is a problem requiring treatment.

In general, real and physiologic ED usually is related to problems with the nerve supply to the penis (e.g., with diabetes, or after some prostate surgeries or prostate radiation), the blood circulation into the penis (impaired in heart failure or sometimes due to a blockage in the pudendal artery, or other major artery supplying blood to the penis), problems with the veins which must trap and keep blood inside the penis to allow the engorgement to make an erection, or failure to get the proper stimulus from the brain (must be relaxed and sexually aroused). If there is something interfering with any or all of these conditions, a full erection will be prevented. If you never wake up with an erection, this may be a sign that there is a physiologic cause of your ED.

Thus, ED can be caused by many and varied problems, including atherosclerosis (hardening of the arteries) or venous leakage (weak veins), nerve diseases due to diabetes, prostate surgery, prolonged bicycle riding on those hard bicycle seats, psychological factors, such as stress, depression, and performance anxiety, as well as physical injury to the penis.

For people who are at risk of developing ED due to personal behavior, such as drinking too much alcohol, steps may be taken to prevent it. Smoking increases a man's chances of developing ED by 50%. Approximately 200 prescribed drugs are known to cause or contribute to ED. However, other causes of ED may not be preventable or easily treatable.

Tips to Improve Erectile Dysfunction

One of the key factors leading to good erectile function is vasodilatation of the small blood vessel in the penis (corpus cavernosum) due to the naturally occurring substance called nitric oxide (NO). This chemical is also sometimes referred to as endothelium derived relaxing factor (EDRF). This is a short-lived chemical that relaxes the smooth muscle in the blood vessel wall to allow more blood into the penis. This is basically nature's nitroglycerin. When you get stimulated, a normal and healthy male response is to produce NO. This will begin and then sustain the erection.

Before we talk about "the little blue pill," there are some pearls that I would like to pass on that may enhance your no function and release without having to take the blue pill. For example, fish oils (EPA and DPA) can enhance the production of NO from the lining cells of your blood vessels. 1-2 grams per day of fish oil may be a more natural way to enhance erectile function.

179

Similarly, L-Arginine, is an amino acid precursor for the production of NO. Although there is little solid scientific evidence showing that L-Arginine will cure ED, like fish oils, it may promote NO production, which should improve erectile dysfunction.

Finally, high saturated fats may inhibit NO production. There may be a connection between eating a Big Mac and then not being able to have a good erection. In one study they examined the ability to make NO before and then shortly after eating a Quarter Pounder with cheese. NO production was definitely inhibited, so next time you are thinking, *This is the night*, maybe you should eat sushi and stay away from that greasy cheeseburger. Finally, smoking will inhibit healthy blood vessel function and NO production. Quitting smoking, losing weight, moderate alcohol consumption and strenuous exercise can all contribute to sustaining healthy sexual function late into your 60s 70s and even into the eighth decade.

PILLS TO IMPROVE ERECTILE DYSFUNCTION

If healthy lifestyle choices and fish oil and L-Arginine do not work, it may be important to consult your doctor and move to more aggressive interventions with medications or other therapies. The type of medical specialist who treats ED will depend on the cause of the problem. Based on your family's medical history as well as your own medical history and current health, your doctor may treat you with oral medications, such as Viagra (see below). If this fails, you may need an evaluation by a urologist or a psychologist. There are many different ways erectile dysfunction can be treated, including oral medications, sex therapy, penile injections, suppositories, vacuum pumps, and surgery. Each type of treatment has its own advantages and disadvantages.

We are all familiar by now with the little blue pill. The brand name for this drug is Viagra. These new pills for ED are very effective for most men. More than twenty-million men have been treated with these medications. Viagra was the first approved in the class of drugs called cyclic nucleotide phosphodiesterases (PDE5) inhibitors. These medications are now considered the first line of treatment for erectile dysfunction. The PDE5 inhibitors sildenafil (Viagra), vardenafil (Levitra) and tadalafil (Cialis) are prescription drugs, which are taken orally. How do these pills work?

When you are aroused the healthy cells lining the inside of the blood vessels in the penis release NO. This in turn releases the chemical cyclic GMP, which is what starts the blood vessel dilatation that leads to the erection. Phosphodiesterase (PDE5) constitutes a group of enzymes that promote the destruction of this important blood vessel dilator, cyclic GMP. By inhibiting PDE5, sildenafil, tadalafil and vardenafil, block the breakdown of cGMP, allowing this dilating chemical to stick around longer and boosting NO's ability to make an erection. These drugs are potent and work for most men. If they do not work then you should definitely consult and expert urologist to look for other pathological causes of your erectile dysfunction.

A few other technique and drugs have been shown to have some efficacy. The drug alprostadil in combination with the permeation enhancer DDAIP has been approved in Canada under the brand name Vitaros as a topical cream first line treatment for erectile dysfunction. Another treatment regimen is injection therapy. One of the following drugs is injected into the penis: papaverine, phentolamine, and prostaglandin. There are also vacuum and other mechanical devices and penile implants that have been used in more extreme cases.

It should be noted that the FDA does not recommend alternative or herbal therapies to treat sexual function. There are many different products advertised as herbal Viagra or natural sexual enhancement products, but there are no clinical trials or scientific studies that support the effectiveness of these products for the treatment of erectile dysfunction.

One interesting and relatively new discovery in this area is that men with atherosclerosis (hardening of the arteries) can develop a severe blockage of the pudendal artery. This is the main artery supplying blood to the penis. Even more interesting is that by using a stent procedure to reopen the blockage it has now been shown that this treatment (stenting of the pudendal artery) can cure the longstanding erectile dysfunction, in most of these men. So, if you have coronary heart disease of blockage in the leg arteries, and you have ED, you may have a blockage in the pudendal artery that could be fixed and cure your ED. Ask your doctor about this new treatment option.

"Low T" (Testosterone and Men's Health)

Low testosterone has been increasingly recognized as a real clinical syndrome in some men as they age. Testosterone, which is predominantly produced in the testes, will normally drop slowly as men age. Testosterone levels decline steadily after age 40. The decline is relatively small, at an average rate of about 1% to 2% percent per year. By middle age and older, virtually all men experience some decline in testosterone. However, only a small percentage of aging men have levels far below those considered normal for their age. If the testosterone levels drop enough, this can be associated with a syndrome that is not that different form women who go through menopause. This syndrome in men has been referred to as andropause. Unlike a woman's menopause, when estrogen levels plummet over months to very low levels, men's andropause is a gradual decline of testosterone levels over years. The effects of low testosterone can be insidious, even go unnoticed.

This syndrome is characterized by changes in mood (fatigue, irritability, depression, anger), decreased libido (low sex drive) decreased body hair, decreased lean body mass and strength and ability to build skeletal muscle, erectile dysfunction, increased abdominal fat, inability to concentrate, rudimentary breast development (man boobs) and low or zero sperm count. Overall, about two-thirds of men with low testosterone will report symptoms. Many men, however, may have these symptoms but may write them off as, "I guess I am just getting older." If you do not have any of these symptoms it is generally recommended that you do not need to check your testosterone level. There is no evidence that treating asymptomatic men with testosterone provides any benefit.

The other confusing issue is that one or more of these signs or symptoms, such as fatigue or erectile dysfunction, may be experienced by men who do not have low testosterone. However, if you have three or more of the symptoms described above it is probably worth checking with your doctor. The diagnosis can be made with a pretty simple blood test (testosterone level less than

300 nanograms/deciliter). So, if you are over forty to sixty years old and have these issues, it is worth checking.

There has been a lot of increased advertising and publicity about low testosterone. It has become a big business. All of this publicity has led to a somewhat shocking, seventeen-fold increase in the diagnosis and treatment of low testosterone the last decade. When appropriate, low testosterone can be treated by using a daily skin gel, patches worn on the skin, orally disintegrating tablets, or injections. In clinical studies, the majority of men with low testosterone have improved erectile function and sex drive with testosterone replacement. About 10% of men will have no response to treatment, and the long-term effects of testosterone replacement therapy have not been well studied. Clinical trials to evaluate the effects of testosterone replacement are underway. Until then, men with low testosterone symptoms whose blood tests show low testosterone levels will need to make their own decisions regarding treatment with their doctors.

SUMMARY

So, in summary, for men, you are only as old as you look and feel. There are so many things that you can do to maintain a youthful body, spirit, mind, and energy. Follow the Burn Calories skeletal building plan and the Rules of eating. Then take advantage of some of the easy to follow pearls such as statins, fish oil, and

DHT blockade to look and feel young. Remember, it is biological age not chronological age that matters. Get young.

Chapter Nine Key Points: Special Pearls for Men

1) Identify the factors that contribute to you looking or feeling old.

2) Decide which of these are important and follow the pearls to "youth."

3) Weight loss, fitness, and diet will start the transformation to feeling young.

4) Grow hair "while you sleep" by taking finasteride or its equivalent, + other Rx.

5) Take care of your skin to look more youthful. It is OK to use creams and Botox!

6) When you are thinner & "fit" you will look and feel more sexual and potent.

7) Enhance your NO production (nitric oxide for erectile function) with exercise, diet and cholesterol lowering, fish oil, ± L-Arginine, & if necessary Viagra/Cialis, etc.

8) If you have low sex drive or function, check your testosterone level and maybe your pudendal artery.

❧ *Chapter Ten* ❧

For Women Only: How to Stay Young and on Top of Your Game: Life Does Not End at Menopause

Staying Young for Women

O K girls, it is time to talk about the biggest health, fitness and youthfulness issues for women. This is admittedly the hardest chapter in the book for me. I am one short on my X-chromosomes. I think I have some pretty good ideas about the main issues that concern the men, but women are tough. When it comes to aging issues, once again there is some element of "Men are from Mars and Women are from Venus." A woman's perspective and concerns about feeling and looking young are in many cases are very different from a man's.

In order to begin to get insights into those "youth" and health issues most relevant to women I have gone to the source, and have polled dozens of women in their 30s to 60s about what key health and youth issues would be of critical interest to them. In this chapter we will focus on some of the most common health issues affecting women as they age. We will address special issues for women related to weight gain and fitness, referring back to the core messaging in this book as well as exploring how being single or in a relationship may affect your risk of being overweight.

This chapter will address some tough questions about heart health, hormone replacement (menopause), and osteoporosis. We will also touch on sexual issues, and cosmetic issues including breasts, and skin that are of interest to many women in their 30s to 70s. Hopefully some of these issues are going to be relevant and helpful to our female audience, and give you some hope and direction.

It's Not Too Late

A critical issue that needs to be addressed is a feeling of resignation among many middle-aged women. They think, "I am overweight, unattractive, and I like to eat. I am married, and my husband is overweight. We almost never have sex anymore, so who really cares how I look?" "It is not worth making any effort to get thin (ner) and fit. I will just be sedentary and keep eating." "It is hopeless. I will never look anything like those girls on the cover of the fashion magazines."

Many women notice an increase in belly fat as they get older, even if they aren't gaining weight. This may be related to a decreasing level of estrogen, which appears to influence where fat is distributed in the body. The tendency to gain or carry weight around the waist, and have an apple rather than a pear shape can have a genetic component as well. This weight change and distribution can be reversed with great nutrition, high intensity exercise as described in this book and possibly with low dose hormone replacement therapy when indicated. If you give up, you will be feeding this negative self-image. Indeed, it is the concession to a sedentary aging process that contributes to a low self-esteem, major health issues, such as coronary heart disease, and a high rate of depression. Life is not over after menopause. You can have the best years of your life ahead of you if you take great care of yourself. You may have an empty nest, but you can live a full and incredible life.

Here is the first key message of the chapter: *It is not too late.* You can change your attitude, your activity, your eating habits, and transform your body and your health, that will create a new feeling of self-esteem that goes along with these behavioral changes. OK, you may not get the cover of Cosmopolitan, but your husband or boyfriend will take notice. If you are looking for a new boyfriend or husband, this will help as well. You may have the satisfaction of having your husband or significant other observe that other men are noticing you! Then, your husband may actually read this book and join you at the gym. You look better, feel better and now you even have a sex life again. Fun!

Sex, Love and Aging

OK, since I brought it up let's talk a little about the importance of maintaining an active sex life as you age. Whether you are young or old, a great relationship includes a balance between mind, spirit and body. As we grow older, our bodies change. Interestingly, two large studies have found that married women, and particularly those with a poor relationship with their husband, tend to gain significantly more weight as they age than single women. Married men also gain more than their single counterparts, but the differential is less, than with married women.

So, as you age, have hormonal changes, gain weight, and lose your body self-esteem it is natural for many couples to lose interest in sex. This is a bad thing. As Dr. Ruth points, "Sex is the glue that holds a relationship together." It is also a highly favored and a fun way to Burn Calories While You Sweat.

If one or both partners are sexually frustrated, this can wreak havoc on the relationship. The couple may be snapping at each other over other matters when the real conflict stems from problems in the sexual arena. The more discord there is in a relationship, the less likely it is that the couple is going to want to have sex. This in turn establishes a vicious cycle that causes not only the couple's sex life, but also the relationship, to spiral downward. This sexual disconnect puts marriages at risk of infidelity and/or divorce. For these reasons, it's vital for couples of any age to be proactive and to keep the fires of passion burning. If sexual fires become completely extinguished, slowly but surely most relationships will die out too.

The good news is that regardless of the reasons for a sexual falling out, excellent help is available. The path of getting thin and fit as outlined in this book may help to reverse the loss of interest in a sex life. It is not the whole answer but a good place to start. When you get thin (or thinner), fit and energized, ideally with your partner in tow, you may be amazed how this can rekindle the sexual part of your life. Make sure the man in your life also reads about the tips in the men's chapter.

Menopause and Hormones

Let's face it. Menopause is challenging for most women. Yes, it is great not having a period to deal with, but the hot flashes, mood swings, effects on skin, weight, etc. are tough to deal with.

In the old days, most women with (natural) postmenopausal symptoms were treated with hormone replacement therapy, using estrogen and progestin, a man-made version of progesterone. Women who had menopause as the result of a hysterectomy would take estrogen alone. This hormone replacement therapy would predictably reduce or eliminate many of the bad side effects of menopause. Hormone therapy was also thought to have the long-term benefits of preventing heart disease and osteoporosis.

Unfortunately, a large study in 2002 demonstrated that routine and lifelong hormone replacement for postmenopausal women may make you feel better, but actually may pose more health risks than benefits. As the number of health hazards attributed to hormone therapy, including an increased risk of breast cancer, uterine cancer (with estrogen without progestin), and possibly coronary heart disease grew, doctors became less likely to prescribe it. Many women taking hormone therapy discontinued its use, often without consulting with their doctors.

Despite its risks, there may also be benefit from hormone therapy for some women. Some physicians still believe that it is appropriate to give at least short-term hormone replacement with estrogen to relieve severe hot flash symptoms. This treatment may have additional benefits including: 1) It may ease vaginal symptoms of menopause, such as dryness, itching, burning and discomfort with intercourse. 2) It may reduce the risk of osteoporosis and hip fractures, 3) It may reduce the risk of colorectal cancer, and 4) Estrogen may decrease risk of heart disease when taken early in your postmenopausal years.

What are the risks of hormone therapy? In the largest clinical trial to date, the combination estrogen-progestin increased

193

the risk of certain serious conditions. According to the study, women taking estrogen plus progestin might experience a slight increase in risk of heart disease, breast cancer, blood clots, stroke and abnormal mammograms than women taking a placebo. The study found no increased risk of breast cancer or heart disease among women taking estrogen without progestin. Over one year, however, estrogen therapy alone was associated with a slight increase in risk of stroke, blood clots, and mammogram abnormalities, than observed in women taking placebo.

So when is hormonal therapy appropriate and acceptably safe? Despite the health risks, estrogen is still the standard for treating menopausal symptoms. The absolute risk to an individual woman taking hormone therapy is quite low and may be low enough to be acceptable to many women, depending on your symptoms.

The benefits of short-term hormone therapy may outweigh the risks if you experience moderate to severe hot flashes or other menopausal symptoms, have lost bone mass and either aren't able to tolerate other treatments or aren't benefitting from other treatments. Hormonal replacement may also be indicated for women who have stopped having periods before age forty (premature menopause). Women who experience premature menopause or premature ovarian failure have a lower risk of breast cancer, a higher risk of osteoporosis, and a higher risk of coronary heart disease (CHD) then women who begin menopause at a later age (say fifty-years-old). Thus, in younger women the protective benefits of hormone therapy may outweigh the risks. Each case is different and women should talk with their primary care physician or their gynecologist about the risks and benefits for their individual circumstance.

OSTEOPOROSIS

Osteoporosis, or the weakening of your bones due to a loss of the mineral and calcium content, remains a major health issue for women as they age. Osteoporosis is a significant health issue for nearly fifty million Americans. Nearly 70% of these patients of osteoporosis are women, according to the National Osteoporosis Foundation. This is a bigger problem for women then for men, due to a smaller amount of bone and muscle mass to start, as well as hormonal issues that can lead to faster bone loss in women.

Hip fractures, hunched backs, back pain, and frailty used to be things older women had to accept before doctors knew anything more about osteoporosis. The good news is that osteoporosis is largely preventable and can even now be reversed with medical therapies. Our bodies build up most of bone mass in early adolescence and up until the age of thirty. After this age it is unusual to be able to create additional (new) bone, and the best we can hope for is to continue to be in equilibrium, making as much bone as we break down every day to maintain our calcium and phosphate balance. As one ages, there are eating and activity behaviors that can promote good bone health and help you avoid bone loss and osteoporosis. Even as we age we are capable of repairing bone damage. It is critical, however, to provide your body with adequate calcium consumption, sunlight to make healthy amounts of vitamin D, and weight-bearing physical activity.

You are at increased risk for osteoporosis if you are a women (which you presumably are if you are reading this chapter), and if you are getting older (try to stop that risk factor), and if you are small and have thin-boned frame. Other risk factors include being Caucasian or Asian, a positive family history of osteoporosis, anorexia, menopause with its associated loss of estrogen, diet low in calcium and/or vitamin D, smoking, sedentary lifestyle and excessive alcohol.

There are a number of relatively simple measures that will reduce your risks of developing clinically important osteoporosis. The main ways to prevent osteoporosis include making sure that you are ingesting adequate amounts of calcium and vitamin D, and that you are physically active with good weight bearing activity. This will include the kind of weight lifting outlined in the Burn

Calories workout as well as other weight bearing activities, including walking, jogging, playing racket sports, skiing, dancing, etc. The role of hormone replacement therapy is touched on in the former section about menopause.

Finally, there are now a number of FDA-approved medications that will help to prevent, or reverse osteoporosis. Many of these agents are in the class of drugs called bisphosphonates. These would include Actonel, Atelvia, Boniva, Fosamax, and Zometa. Bisphosphonates are drugs that inhibit mineralization or resorption of the bone by blocking the action of osteoclasts, which are the cells that break down the mineral content in the bone. Other drugs also have been shown to retard or help prevent osteoporosis, including thiazide diuretics, calcitonin (Fortical) and various estrogen agonists including Climara, Evista, Premarin, Vivelle and others.

More recently, the Food and Drug Administration approved the drug Prolia (denosumab) for use in treating osteoporosis in postmenopausal women. The drug works by preventing the breakdown and re-absorption of bone and calcium, thereby letting bone growth catch up to bone loss. Unlike some of the other osteoporosis medications, Prolia is injected by a doctor every six months, in part to ensure patients do not miss any daily doses and to be more convenient than a daily or weekly regimen.

So, in summary, there are numerous ways that women can reduce their risk of morbidity from osteoporosis. These include proper diet, calcium intake and weight bearing exercise, as well as additional medications when appropriate. It is beyond the scope of this book to provide exact recommendations for individual patients. It is suggested that you consult with your primary physician and/or gynecologist for specific guidelines and recommendations for you.

COSMETIC SURGERY

"Beauty is more important than health." That is what one of my close—and very intelligent—women friends told me when I asked her about women's issues related to aging. The focus on beauty, even if it requires invasive procedures or major surgery, has accelerated in the last twenty years.

Indeed, the fastest growing consumer group for surgical and nonsurgical cosmetic enhancement procedures is middle-aged women (40-55 years). Experts cite appearance evaluation (judgmental thoughts of beliefs surrounding the body, and body dissatisfaction) and appearance investment (i.e., how much a person's self-worth is dependent upon appearance) as two major factors in choosing to have plastic surgery. Western cultural norms equate aging with a loss of physical attractiveness, so it is natural that women experience aging anxiety as they perceive they are becoming less attractive as they age.

At the same time, the media has increased public awareness of cosmetic surgery and has placed pressure on aging women (and men) to have wrinkle-free faces. The increased exposure to cosmetic surgery in the media has normalized plastic surgery as an acceptable method of addressing issues of body dissatisfaction. Some people believe that this is a symptom of underlying psychological issues at both an individual and societal level.

For women, the appearance of your skin is very important to youth-fullness. Having great skin is partly genetic but also very dependent on key environmental and behavioral issues. The most critical factors include smoking, which causes lack of blood flow to the skin and major aging, as well as sun/ultraviolet exposure which also causing recurring skin damage and aging. If you care about your skin, don't smoke. If you care about your skin, do not lay out in the sun, frying like a donut in baby oil.

Avoid the sun, wear a hat and use sunscreen. Unfortunately, tanning booths with high levels of ultraviolet light exposure are also a no-no if you want to avoid a facelift at age forty, or worse. Much of the aging caused by over-exposure to the sun and tanning booths cannot be erased by cosmetic surgery. In addition to the cosmetic risks of sun exposure, the increasing focus on being tanned year round is also correlated with a rising incidence of the deadly cancer, melanoma, in women. In fact, melanoma is the most common form of cancer in women between the ages of twenty-five and twenty-nine and its incidence has tripled in women under forty in the last thirty years. So, the bottom line is—limit your ultraviolet exposure for youthful skin and cancer prevention.

How about other measures to reduce or prevent wrinkles? Almost everyone knows about botox (botulinum toxin). As mentioned in the section for men, it is expensive and a little painful, but it works. This is a neurotoxin that essentially paralyzes some of the small muscles in your face and reduces the effects of those muscles in causing wrinkles. This is particularly effective in the wrinkles of the forehead. It also can help with other small wrinkles, like at the corners of the eyes (crow's feet), etc. It is a prescription treatment. Although there is a little pain with the injections, the main pain is to your wallet. To be effective, the treatments need to be given once every 3-4 months initially. If you are interested in this investment in your skin, you should probably start in your 30s or 40s. After a few years the intervals may expand out to only once every 5-6 months. This is not for everyone. However, it is one of the most effective ways, short of plastic surgery, to reduce the effects of aging on your skin.

What if you are past the "Botox" stage? You have a lot of excess, wrinkles and skin around your eyes, or forehead or neck and chin. Cosmetic surgery can be very effective for this, but it is painful both physically and financially. It is also very dependent on finding a great plastic surgeon. There is nothing worse than spending a lot of money, suffering a lot of pain and then getting a bad result or having serious surgical complications. So do your homework and go to a reputable surgeon, if not the best in your region, if you can afford it.

How about other cosmetic surgery? It is also beyond the scope of this book to go into depth about all of the cosmetic surgery options that can be individualized for you specific needs. Popular options for many women include, liposuction to remove cellulite, "tummy tucks" and breast revisions to reduce fat or skin in the abdominal area or breasts, which may be important option to consider if you have lost a lot of weight and have sagging and excess skin. Again, these can be pretty major surgeries, depending on your specific needs.

Finally, a few words about breast implants. This remains one of the most popular plastic surgery procedures. There are two main types of breast implants now available to women: saline and silicone. Saline implants are filled with saline, usually at the time of surgery. Saline implants have been criticized for feeling hard or unnatural, but improved surgical techniques have lessened these complaints. Silicone implants are pre-filled with silicone gel, a thick, sticky fluid that mimics the feel of human fat. Some women feel that silicone breast implants look and feel more like natural breast tissue than their saline counterparts.

Breast implant surgery is not totally benign either in cost, or medical risks. The risks of breast implant surgery include the potential for permanent changes in nipple or breast sensation, infection, implant leakage or rupture, scar tissue that encases the implant and makes the breast distorted and firm, as well as the potential need for additional breast revision surgeries. Breast implants may also interfere with breast cancer screening. Although it may be easier to see or feel breast lumps if you have breast implants, the implants may complicate routine mammography to screen for breast cancer. You may need additional images offering special views of your breasts, and the images may be harder to interpret because cancers can be obscured by the implants. Finally, breast implants may hamper breast-feeding.

The biggest decision, of course, is whether or not to get breast implants. For some women this can be very positive, and can raise their self-esteem. They think they will be more attractive with large breasts. Without dwelling on this or being judgmental, I believe that many women undergo this procedure for the wrong reasons and sometimes with misperceptions about what men like and the potential risks.

When polled, a significant majority of men do not like very large breasts. This may be shocking to some women, but it is true. Even more interesting and potentially relevant are the surveys that show that a large majority of men do not like women with breast implants. So if most men do not like very large breasts, and an even larger majority of men prefer natural to breast implants, it may be important to examine your own personal reasons for having this done, prior to signing up for breast implant surgery. Each woman and each case must be thought out carefully. This can be a very positive intervention for some women. For example, if you are married and your husband thinks it will make you much more attractive, maybe it would be worth it. If you are single and have B cup size or larger breasts, that are proportional to your body type, you may want to reconsider. In the end it is a very personal decision, but not a trivial one.

HEART DISEASE AND WOMEN

We hear a lot about breast cancer, but three times as many women die from heart disease than from breast cancer. In women, the condition is responsible for nearly 30% of deaths, as reported by the CDC. Heart disease is the leading killer of both men and women, and contrary to common belief, more women than men die from heart disease each year.

More than 470,000 American women lose their lives each year as a result of heart attacks, strokes, and other cardiovascular diseases. In fact, more women than men die from heart disease each year. Women are generally protected from coronary heart disease until menopause. Estrogen and progesterone provide protection, perhaps through their effects on cholesterol, and especially the effects in raising the good cholesterol (HDL) for younger women. Unfortunately, after menopause this protection begins to fade, HDL levels generally drop and women begin to quickly catch up with the men in their 60s and 70s. Women who smoke have high blood pressure and type 2 diabetes from obesity are now presenting at younger and younger ages with heart attacks. So even younger women are not necessarily immune from heart disease if they ignore conventional risk factors.

Until recently, little research focused on women and heart disease, but the good news is that's no longer the case. From research into the effects of hormone replacement therapy on heart health to studies of how cholesterol-lowering medications work in women, there's an unprecedented increase in the amount of information available to women working to live with and prevent heart disease.

Again, the complete approach to heart and vascular disease for women is beyond the scope of this book. However, we will touch on the key issues. If you are a woman and do not want to die from, or have the morbidity from a stroke or heart attack you will, like men, need to address some basic behavioral issues. First, don't smoke. Eat a diet low in fat and rich in fruits, vegetables, whole grains, and low-fat dairy products, exercise at 20-30 minutes, at least 2-3 times/week (ideally as outlined in Chapter Three), to maintain a healthy weight and avoid type 2 diabetes.

In addition, you should see your primary care physician each year for a health examination, including a blood pressure and cholesterol screenings. High blood pressure may affect more than 1/3 of all women over the age of 40. Studies indicate that there is a nearly 50% increase in stroke risk for women for each 7.5 mm Hg increase in their diastolic blood pressure, so monitoring blood pressure and controlling hypertension are critical in avoiding both stroke and heart attacks. Revisit Chapter Seven (Know Your Cholesterol) if you need to be reminded about the critical importance of low lipids in promoting cardio-vascular health.

Another very important factor in the morbidity and mortality from heart disease in women is related to the failure to diagnose certain atypical presentations in women with coronary disease. Women may often present with funny chest pains, arm or neck pains, headaches, generalized fatigue, or mild shortness of breath rather than typical chest tightness with exertion. All too often this results in a late or incorrect diagnosis. In women, the symptoms caused by coronary artery blockage, or even a full-blown heart attack may be missed by both the doctor and the patient. Although the stereotypical heart attack patient is a middle aged male, women are at high risk as they age, particularly if they have not paid attention to their risk factors (smoking, hypertension, high cholesterol, diabetes and family history).

Psychological Well-Being and Depression for Women

Depression is a frequent issue in our society, but affects more women than men. Approximately twelve-million women are affected by a depressive disorder each year, compared to about six-million men. Studies have found that married women and mothers are especially vulnerable to depression. Depression is both chemical and environmental, in most cases. The risk factors for developing depression include, a family history of depression, hormonal changes (particularly after pregnancy with a huge drop in hormone levels), serious chronic illness, heart problems, serious problems in your relationship with your husband or significant other, stressful life events such as the death of a loved one or loss of job, substance abuse, certain medications that can promote or trigger depression, vitamin or thyroid deficiencies, as well as other various conditions including anxiety or eating disorders.

The best way to prevent depression for women, as well as men, is to create a social network that includes friends, family and in most cases a good relationship with a significant other. The least depressed and healthiest adults, both in women and men, are people in significant caring relationships. However, if you are not in a close and nurturing relationship you can reduce your risk of depression by making efforts to reach out into the community. It is very important to find a purpose and meaningful reason to get up each morning. Work, community service, love, pets, and volunteering are great things to look forward to each day.

Depression is treatable. It is important for a woman who feels she may be suffering from depression to be carefully evaluated by a physician because the source of the depressive symptoms could be birth control pills, hormone replacement therapy, or thyroid disease. Treatment for depression, like most other psychological conditions, may include psychotherapy and/or medication. There may be many other complementary approaches that may include meditation, group counseling, etc.

Importantly, strenuous physical exercise can also be a great antidepressant. Following the high intensity workout strategy outlined in this book, combined with proper eating will be very helpful. If you can adopt these lifestyle changes, and change your fitness and lose weight to closer to your ideal body weight it is likely that you will begin to feel much better about yourself, and gain self-esteem. This will often translate into other great improvements in your life including attracting or holding onto a significant other, getting a new job, having a better sex life. All of these changes will promote better mental health and start you on a path to be less depressed and more confident about yourself, and your life.

Summary

So, in summary, for women, just like men, you are only as old as you look and feel. There are so many things that you can do to maintain a youthful body, spirit, mind, and energy. Follow the Burn Calories skeletal muscle building plan and the Rules of eating. Then take advantage of some of the easy to follow pearls such as appropriate use of hormone therapy, selective use of cosmetic surgery to touch–up key cosmetic areas, and pay attention to your significant other, including an active sex life, to maintain or improve your mental health and feel young. Remember, it is biological age not chronological age that matters. Be young.

Chapter Ten Key Points: Special Pearls for Women

1) Identify the factors that contribute to you looking or feeling old.

2) Decide which of these are important and follow the pearls to "youth".

3) Weight loss, fitness, and diet will start the transformation to feeling young.

4) Take care of your skin to look more youthful. Avoid the sun and use sunscreen.

5) Hormone replacement therapy may be appropriate for some women.

6) Selective use of cosmetic procedures to enhance your looks and self-esteem.

7) Weight bearing exercise, vitamin D and drugs to prevent osteoporosis.

8) Remember that women are not immune to heart disease! Know your cholesterol.

9) Pay attention to significant other, family, friends and community to stay mentally engaged, youthful and avoid depression.

❧ *Chapter Eleven* ❧

Epilogue: Looking Great, and Feeling Great, Living Longer

I never promised you a rose garden, and I never said that the results achievable via the methods outlined in this book could be accomplished without some initial pain and commitment. It does require a new mindset and the motivation to change your body and your life for the better. I promise you that the highly efficient approach to exercise and eating that is outlined in this book will lead to success. If you can commit to 30-40 minutes of high intensity muscle stress, 2-3 times per week with aerobic, circuit weight training, crunches in your car, isometric fidgeting, and following the 10 rules of eating, you WILL become much thinner, and fit.

These changes in your lifestyle and your weight and fitness will translate into much greater energy and skeletal muscle strength. This will transform your everyday experiences in life. It will improve your outlook on life, your mood, your relationships, and your sex life. Perhaps most importantly, if you follow and adopt the lifestyle changes in this book you can also expect to live longer, and with a much better quality of your life. If you are 45-50 years old, and a type 2 diabetic with severe high blood pressure, and you sustainably lose 60 pounds using the approach taught in this book, you can cure your diabetes, and drop your blood pressure by 30 points. Statistically, you will have added an average of 5-6 years to your lifespan.

I will come back to the theme and messaging that we emphasized in the early part of the book. It is time to take care of the most important possession in your life. Your body. It is time to value and care for this sacred vehicle of your life and health. It is time to care more about the health and fitness of your body than the shine on your car or the song playlist on your iPod. It is time to transform your experience of life.

It is time to achieve what I have achieved using this approach. Yes at age 40 or 50 or even 60, you can get back to your high school graduation weight and be twice as strong as you were at age 20. It may sound crazy, but you can do this. And, you can do this without spending 2 hours a day, 6 days a week on the treadmill. That is not the answer. That is burning calories while you sweat, and will not substantially alter your basal metabolic rate to burn calories while you sleep. High intensity, short duration, repetitive skeletal muscle stress will transform your metabolism and allow you to achieve this with the minimum time commitment possible. This is highly efficient. It is specifically targeted for the super-busy, multitasking adults of our generation.

Eating correctly is a crucial part of this plan. Post a copy of the ten rules of eating on your refrigerator. Read the rules every morning until you can recite them by memory to your friends and loved ones. Teach these rules to your children! Most importantly, embed these rules in your conscious and subconscious mind. Do not eat when you are not hungry. Stop eating when you are full. Eat small meals 4-5 times per day and slow down your eating. Get those processed carbohydrates, sugar-rich and fried foods out of you everyday diet! Weigh yourself every day and close the loop, to get the positive feedback that you will see over time as you make these relatively modest and highly efficient lifestyle changes.

Stop watching and buying into the quick, easy infomercial fixes. The gimmicky, fad, diets and the DVDs with exercise plans designed for top NFL athletes is not the right plan for you. It is too hard, and it is not necessary to achieve the fitness and weight loss and longevity that you are looking for. These fad programs do not work well and are not sustainable. Empty your closet of the exercise bands, ab dominators, easy glides, and all the other junk that you have bought from those infomercials, expecting a quick fix.

Know your cholesterol. If you do not know it, get it checked with your doctor or your local health clinic. If your LDL is above 100 or your ratio (total cholesterol/HDL) is greater than 3.5, you need to do something about your cholesterol. Diet and exercise will help but it may not be enough. You may need to start on a medication like a statin (every second or third day may be adequate) to reduce your LDL cholesterol, and reduce your risk of heart attack or stroke. Know your blood pressure as well. If you are hypertensive at age fifty and do not get treated you can expect a five-year reduction, on the average, in your life expectancy.

Importantly, the great killers of sedentary and overweight adults are high cholesterol, high blood pressure, type 2 diabetes (from obesity), and smoking. All of these risk factors that will dramatically shorten your life expectancy and decrease your quality of life (other than the smoking) are pretty directly related to overeating, under-metabolizing and being obese. If you follow the rules of eating and exercising outlined in this book you will lose weight and be fit. You will cure your hypertension and obesity. You will lower your cholesterol and increase your good cholesterol (HDL). You will feel better, younger, stronger, healthier and have more energy. You will live longer.

We said this at the beginning of the book, and it is worth repeating one last time. If these benefits can be achieved very

213

simply and efficiently to make you look better, feel better and live longer, I hope that the huge rewards will motivate a large percentage of the readers. If you got this far, you did not give up and sell or give this book to a friend. You read it. Now it is time to live it, and to live longer. I have a lot of faith in the human spirit. I have a lot of faith in the ability of people to change their lifestyle when they know that their health, the quality of their life and longevity depend on it. You can follow these simple changes in your life. You can change your metabolism and burn calories while you sleep. You can be thin and fit, and live a better and a longer life. You should teach and model all of these new behaviors for your children, to put an end to the obesity epidemic in America. I wish everyone great success, and the determination to make these changes. Good luck and great health to all.

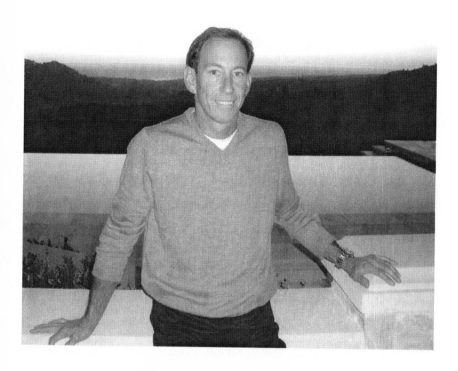

❧ About the Author ❧

D r. Tim Alexander Fischell is a well-known interventional cardiologist, inventor, and serial medical device entrepreneur. He has had a long-standing interest in health and fitness.

After graduating from Cornell University, in Ithaca New York, he attended Cornell University Medical College, in New

York City and received his M.D. degree in 1981. His interest in adult medicine and health led to his decision to pursue a career in internal medicine and cardiology. He completed his internal medicine training at the Massachussetts General Hospital (Harvard University), and then did his cardiology fellowship training at Stanford University, in Palo Alto, California. After his training, he joined the full-time teaching faculty at the Stanford University Medical Center. He was recruited to Nashville, TN to be the Director of the Cardiac Catheterization Laboratories and Director of interventional cardiology at Vanderbilt University in 1992.

For the past fifteen years he has served as Director of Cardiovascular Research at the Borgess Medical Center in southwest Michigan, and is a Professor of Medicine at Michigan State University. He is a serial inventor and entrepreneur, being co-inventor of the heart stent for Johnson and Johnson, an implantable heart attack detector (Angel Medical Systems), and most recently a new catheter invention to treat high blood pressure. He has published more than 120 peer-reviewed scientific papers and book chapters.

He is known for his dedication to his patients' health and well-being. As a cardiologist he has dealt, over decades, with his heart patients' struggles with weight problems, high blood pressure, and diabetes. In the Burn Calories project, he has used his creative spirit, and his caring and passion for patient care to focus his efforts to develop a sustainable approach to help adults deal with the physical challenges of getting healthy, fit, and thin as they age. He is excited to share his inventive health concepts with the readers of this book.

Acknowledgement

My thanks to Dr. Mazen Roumia, for his efforts and contribution to the background research.

References

Folsom AR, Kaye SA, Sellers TA, Hong CP, Cerhan JR, Potter JD, Prineas RJ.

Body fat distribution and 5-year risk of death in older women. JAMA Jan. 27, 1993; 269:4.

Després JP, Lemieux I. Abdominal obesity and metabolic syndrome. Nature Dec. 14, 2006, Vol 444:14.

Després JP. Health consequences of visceral obesity. Ann Med 2001; 33:534-541.

Muggeo M, Verlato G, Bonora E, Bressan F, Girotto S, Borbellini M, Gemma

ML, Moghetti R, Zenere M, Cacciatori V, Zoppini G, DeMarco R. The Verona diabetes study: a population-based survey on known diabetes mellitus prevalence and 5-year all-cause mortality. Diabetologia 1995, 38:318-325.

Hauner H, Stangl K, Schmatz C, Burger K, Blömer H, Pfeiffer EF. Body fat distribution in men with angiographically confirmed coronary artery disease. Atherosclerosis, 1990, 85:203-210.

Klein S, Burke LE, Bray GA, Blair S, Allison DB, Pi-Sunyer X, Hong Y, Eckel RH. Clinical implications of obesity with specific focus on cardiovascular disease. A statement for professionals from the American Heart Association council on nutrition, physical activity, and metabolism. Circulation 2004; 110:2952-2967.

Nakamura T, Tokunaga K, Shimomura I, Nishida M, Yoshida S, Kotani K, Islam AHMW, Keno Y, Kobatake T, Nagai Y, Fujioka S, Tarui S, Matsuzawa Y. Contribution of visceral fat accumulation to the development of coronary artery disease in non-obese men. Atherosclerosis 1994; 107:239-246.

Onat A, Uyarel Hüseyin U, Hergene G, Karabulut A, Albayrak S, Can G. Determinants and definition of abdominal obesity as related to risk of diabetes, metabolic syndrome and coronary disease in Turkish men: A prospective cohort study. Atherosclerosis 2007; 191:182-190.

Vajo Z, Terry JG, Brinton A. Increased intra-abdominal fat may lower HDL levels by increasing the fractional catabolic rate of Lp A-I in postmenopausal women. Atherosclerosis 2002; 160:495-501.

Lakka TA, Lakka HM, Salonen R, Kaplan GA, Salonen JT. Atherosclerosis 2001;154:497-504.

Nissen SE, Nicholls SJ, Wolski K; et al. JAMA 2008; 299(13):1547-1560.

Steinberger J, Daniels SR. Circulation 2003; 107:1448-1453.

Bruen C. Variation of basal metabolic rate per unit surface area with age. The Journal of General Physiology April 8, 1930; 607-616.

Van Pelt RE, Jones PP, Davey KP, DeSouza CA, Tanaka H, Davy BM, Seals DR. J. Clin. Endocrinol. Metab. 1997 82:3208-3212.

Johnstone AM, Murison SD, Duncan JS, Rance KA, Speakman JR. Factors influencing variation in basal metabolic rate include fat-free mass, fat mass, age, and circulating thyroxine but not sex, circulating leptin, or triiodothyronine. Am J Clin Nutr 2005; 82:941-8.

Van Pelt RE, Dinneno FA, Seals DR, Jones PP. Age-related decline in RMR in physically active men: relation to exercise volume and energy intake. J. Clin.Endocrinol. Metab 2001; 281:633-639.

Fukagawa NK, Bandini LG, Young JB. Effect of age on body composition and resting metabolic rate. JAMA 1993 vol 269, No. 4.

Moe B, Angelier F, Beck C, Chastel O. Is basal metabolic rate influenced by age in a long-lived seabird, the snow petrel? The Journal of Experimental Biology 2007; 210: 3407-3414.

Lazzer S, Bedogni G, Lafortuna CL, Marazzi N, Busti C, Galli R, DeCol A, Agosti F, Sartorio A. Relationship between basal metabolic rate, gender, age, and body composition in 8,780 white obese subjects. Obesity2009; 18:71-78.

Baumgartner RN, Waters DL, Gallagher D, Morley JE, Garry PJ. Predictors of skeletal muscle mass in elderly men and women. Mechanisms of Ageing and Development 1999; 107:123-136.

Thomas DR. Sarcopenia. Clin Geriatr Med. 2010; 26:331-346.

Aloia JF, Vaswani A, Feuerman M, Mikhail M, Ma, R. differences in skeletal and muscle mass with aging in black and white women. Am J Physiol Endocrinol Metab 2000; 278:E1153-E1157.

Prior SJ, Roth SM, Wang X, Kammerer C, Miljkovic-Gacic I, Bunker Ch, Wheeler VW,Patrick Al, Zmuda JM. Genetic and environmental influences on skeletal muscle phenotypes as a function of age and sex in large, multigenerational families of African heritage. J Appl Physiol 2007; 103:1121-1127.

Speakman JR, Westerterp KR. Associations between energy demands, physical activity, and body composition in adult humans between 18 and 96 years of age. Am J Clin Nautr 2010; 92:826-834.

Hughes VA, Frontera WR, Roubenoff R, Evans WJ, Fiatarone Singh MA. Longitudinal changes in body composition in older men and women: role of body weight changes and physical activity. Am J Clin Nutr2002; 76:473-481.

Kent-Braun JA, NG AV. Skeletal muscle oxidative capacity in young and older women and men. J Appl Physiol 2000'89:1072-1078.

Larsen RG, Callahan DM, Foulis SA, Kent-Braun JA. In vivo oxidative capacity varies with muscle and training status in young adults. J Appl Physiol 2009; 107:873-879.

Coggan AR, Abduljalil AM, Swanson SC, Earle MS, Farris JW, Mendenhall LA, Robitaille PM. Muscle metabolism during exercise in young and older untrained and endurance-trained Men. J Appl Physiol 1993; 75(5):2125-2133.

King DS, Dalsky GP, Staten MA, Clutter WE, Van Houten DR, Holloszy JO. Insulin action and secretion in endurance-trained humans. J Appl Physiol 1987; 63(6); 2247-2252.

Chilibeck PD, Paterson DH, Smith WDF, Cunningham DA. Cardio-respiratory kinetics during exercises of different muscle groups mass in old and young. J Appl Physiol 1996; 81(3):1388-1394.

Coggan AR, Raguso CA, Williams BD, Sidossis LA, Gastaldelli A. Glucose kinetics during high-intensity exercise in endurance-trained and untrained humans. J Appl Physiol1995; 78(3):1203-1207.

Chad KE, Quigley BM. Exercise intensity: effect on post exercise O2 uptake in trained and untrained women. J Appl Physiol 1991; 70(4):1713-1719.

Thomas TR, Londeree BR, Gerhardt KO, Gehrke CW. Fatty acid profile and cholesterol in skeletal muscle of trained and untrained men. J Appl Physiol 1977; 43(4):709-713.

Zoladz JA, Korzeniewski B, Grassi B. Training-induced acceleration of oxygen uptake kinetics in skeletal muscle: the underling mechanisms. Journal of Physiology and Pharmacology 2006; 57, Suppl 10:67-84.

Zouhal Hassane, Jacob C, Delamarche P, Gratas-Delamarche A. Catecholamine's and the effects of exercise, training and gender. Sports Med 2008'38(5):401-423.

Short KR, Sedlock DA. Excess post exercise oxygen consumption and recovery rate in trained and untrained subjects. J Appl Physiol 1997; 83(4):153-159.

Kalliokoski KK, Knuuti J, Nuutila P. Relationship between muscle blood flow and oxygen uptake during exercise in endurance-trained and untrained men. J Appl Physiol 2005; 98:380-383.

Korzeniewski B, Zoladz JA. Training-induced adaptation of oxidative phosphorylation in skeletal muscles. Biochem, J 2003; 374:37-40.

Kuk JL, Lee S, Heymsfield SB, Ross R. Waist circumference and abdominal adipose tissue distribution: influence of age and sex.Am J Clin Nutr 2005; 81:1330-1334.

Balkau B, Deanfield JE, Després, Bassand JP, fox KAA, Smith SC, Barter P,Tan CE, Gaal LV, Wittchen HU, Massien C, Haffner SM. International day for the evaluation of abdominal obesity (IDRA) A study of waist circumference, cardiovascular disease, and diabetes mellitus in 168,000 primary care patients in 63 countries. Circulation 2007'116:1942-1951.

Delzenne N, Blundell J, Brouns F, Cunningham k, De Graal K, Erkner A, Lluch A, Mars M, Peters HPF, Westerterp-Plantenga M. Gastrointestinal targets of appetite regulation in humans. Obesity reviews 2010; 11:234-250.

Ahima RS, Antwi DA. Brain regulation of appetite and satiety. Endocrinol Metab Clin North Am. 2008; 37(4):811-823.

Marciani L, Gowland PA, Spiller RC, Manoj P, et al... Effect of meal viscosity and nutrients on satiety, intragastric dilution and emptying assessed by MRI. Am J Physiology 2001; 280(6):G1227-1233.

Goetze O, Steingoetter A, Menne D, van der Voort IR, Kwiatek MA, Boesiger P, Weishaupt D, Thumshirn M, Fried M, Schwizer W. Am J Physiol Gastrointest Liver Physiol 2007; 292:G11-G17.

Geliebter A. Gastric distension and gastric capacity in relation to food intake in humans. Physiology & Behavior 1988; 44:665-668.

Oesch S, Rüegg C, Fischer B, Degen L, Beglinger. Effect of gastric distension prior to eating on food intake and feelings of satiety in humans. Physiology & Behavior2006'87:903-910.

Andrews JM, Doran S, Hebbard GS, Rassias G, Sun WM, Horowitz M. Effect of glucose supplementation on appetite and the pyloric motor response to intraduodenal glucose and lipid. Am J Physiol Gastrointest Liver Physiol 1998; 274:645-652.

Niwano Y, Adachi T, Kashimura AJ, Sakata T, Sasaki H, Sekine K, Yamamoto S, Yonekubo A, Kimura S. Is glycemic index of food a feasible predictor of appetite, hunger, and satiety? J Nutr Sci Vitaminol 2009; 55:201-207.

Kwiatek MA, Menne D, Steingoetter An, Goetze O, Forras-Kaufman Z, Kaufman E, Fruehauf H, Boesiger P, Fried M, Schwier W, Fox MR. Effect of meal volume and calorie load on postprandial gastric function and emptying: studies under physiological conditions by combined fiber-optic pressure measurement and MRI. Am J Physiol Gastrointest Liver Physiol 2009; 297:G894-G901.

Berry MK, Russo A, Wishart JM, Tonkin A, Horowitz M, Jones KL. Effect of solid meal on gastric emptying of, and glycemic and cardiovascular responses to, liquid glucose in older subjects. Am J Physiol Gastrointest Liver Physiol 2003; 284: G655-G662.

Expert Panel as Appendix A. clinical Guidelines on the identification, evaluation, and treatment of overweight and obesity in adults: executive summary. Am J Clin Nutr 1998; 68:899-917.

Ball SD, Keller KR, Moyer-Mileur LJ, Ding YW, Donaldson D, Jackson D. Prolongation of satiety after low versus moderately high glycemic index meals in obese adolescents. Pediatrics 2003; 111:488-494.

Lemieux S, Prud'homme D, Moorjani S, Tremblay A, Bouchard C, Lupien PJ, Després JP. Do elevated levels of abdominal visceral adipose tissue contribute to age-related differences in plasma lipoprotein concentrations in men? Atherosclerosis 1995; 118:155-164.

Rexrode KM, Carey VJ, Hennekens CH, et al. Abdominal adiposity and coronary heart disease in women. JAMA 1998; 280 :(21)1843-1848.

Després JP, Lemieux I. Abdominal obesity and metabolic syndrome. Nature 2006; 444:881-887.

Choi SY, Kim D, Oh BH, Kim M, Park HE, Lee CH, Cho SH. General and abdominal obesity and abdominal visceral fat accumulation associated with coronary artery calcification in Korean men. Atherosclerosis 2010; 213:273-278.

Rader DJ. Effect of insulin resistance, dyslipidemia, and intra-abdominal adiposity on the development of cardiovascular disease and diabetes mellitus. The American Journal of Medicine 2007; Vol. 120(3A):S12-S18.

Khan SE, Hull RL, Utzschneider KM. Mechanisms linking obesity to insulin resistance and type 2 diabetes. Nature 2006; Vol 444:840-846.

Khan BB, Flier JS. Obesity and insulin resistance. The Journal of Clinical Investigation 2000; Vol 106(4):473-481.

Caprio S, Bronson M, Sherwin RS, Rife F, Tamborlane WV. Co-existence of severe insulin resistance and hyperinsulinaemia in pre-adolescent obese children. Diabetologia 1996; 39:1489-1497.

Tataranni PA. Pathophysiology of obesity-induced insulin resistance and type 2 diabetes mellitus. Eur Rev Med Pharmacol Sci 2002; 6:27-32.

Qatanani M, Lazar MA. Mechanisms of obesity-association insulin resistance: many choices on the menu. Genes Dev. 2007; 21:1443-1455.

Kelly DE, Goodpaster BH. Skeletal muscle triglyceride. Diabetes Care 2001; 24:933-941.

Petersen KF, Shulman GI. Etiology of insulin resistance. The American Journal of Medicine 2006; Vol 119(5A):105-165.

Boden G. Free fatty acids, insulin resistance, and type 2 diabetes mellitus. Proc Assoc Am Physicians 1999 May-June; 11(3):241-248.

DeFronzo RA. Insulin resistance, lipotoxicity, type 2 diabetes and atherosclerosis: the missing links. The Claude Bernard lecture 2009. Diabetologia 2010; 52:1270-1287.

Kelley DE, Mandarino LJ. Fuel selection in human skeletal muscle in insulin resistance. Diabetes 2000; 49:677-683.

Fujimoto T, Kemppainen J, Kalliokoski KK, Muutila P, Ito M, Knuuti J. Skeletal muscle glucose uptake response to exercise in trained and untrained men. Med Sci Sports Exerc 2003; 35(5):777-783.

Halton TL, Hu FB. The effects of high protein diets on thermogenesis, satiety and weight loss: a critical review. Journal of the American College of Nutrition, 2004; 23(5):373-385.

Rothblum ED. Women and weight: Fad and fiction. The Journal of Psychology1990; 124(1):5-24.

Allen S. Cholesterol: What Camp are you in? Nutritional Perspectives: Journal of the council on Nutrition of the American Chiropractic Ass. 2006; 29(1):23-27.

Balart LA. Diet options of obesity: Fad or famous? Gastroenterol Clin N Am 2005'34:83-9.

Anderson JW, Konz EC, Jenkins DJA. Health advantages and disadvantages of weight-reducing diets: A computer analysis and critical review. Journal of the American College of Nutrition 2000; 19(5):578-590.

Evenson B. "Smart-drug, smart-food" fad winning converts despite scientists' skepticism. Can Med Assoc j 1993148(4):616-617.

Moyad MA. Fad diets and obesity-Part IV: low-carbohydrate vs. low-fat diets. Urologic Nursing 2005; 25(1):67-70.

Mobley C. Fad diets: Facts for dental professionals. J Am Dent Assoc 2008; 139:48-50.

Braganza SF, Ozuah PO. Fad Therapies. Pediatr Rev2005; 26:371-376.

Daniels J. Fad diets: slim on good nutrition. Nursing 2004 34(12):22-23.

Ness-Abramof R, Apovian CM. Endocrine2006; 29(1):5-9.

Astrup A, Larsen TM, Harper A. Atkins and other low-carbohydrate diets: hoax or an effective tool for weight loss? Lancet 2004; 364:897-899.

Moyad MA. Fad diets and obesity-part II: an introduction to the theory behind low-carbohydrate diets. Urologic Nursing 2004; 24(3):210-213.

Kelley GA, Kelley KS. Aerobic exercise and HDL2 –C: a meta-analysis of randomized controlled trials. Atherosclerosis 2006'184:207-215.

82.Alkerwi A, Boutsen M, Vaillant M, Barre J, Lair ML, Albert A, Guillaume M, Dramaix M. Alcohol consumption and the prevalence of metabolic syndrome; a meta-analysis of observational studies. Atherosclerosis 2009; 204:624-635.

Sharrett AR, Ballantyne CM, Coady SA, Heiss G, Sorlie PD, Catellier D, Patsch W. Coronary heart disease prediction from lipoprotein cholesterol levels, triglycerides, lipoprotein (a), apolipoproteins A-I and B, and HDL density subfractions: the atherosclerosis risk in communities (ARIC) study. Circulation 2001; 104:1108-1113.

Gaziano JM, Buring JE, Breslow JL, Goldhaber SZ, Rosner B, VanDenburgh M, Willett W, Hennekens CH. Moderate alcohol intake, increased levels of high-density lipoprotein and its subfractions, and decreased risk of myocardial infarction. N Engl J Med 1993; 329(25):1830-1834.

DeBacker G. New European guidelines for cardiovascular disease prevention in clinical practice. Clin Chem Lab Med 2009; 47(2):138-142.

Geroldi D, Emanuele E. Moderate alcohol consumption and atherosclerosis: friend or foe? Atheroslerosis 2010; 210:367-368.

Liu Y, Tanaka H, Sasazuki S, Yoshimasu K, Kodama H, Washio M, Tanake K, Tokunaga S, Kono Su, Arai H, Koyanagi S, Hiyamuta K, Doi Y, Kawano T, Nakagaki O, Takada K, Nii T, Shirai K, Ideishi M, Arakawa K, Mohri M, Takeshita A. Alcohol consumption and severity of angiographically determined coronary artery disease in Japanese men and women. Atherosclerosis 2001; 156:177-183.

De Oliveira e Silva ER, Foster D, McGee Harper M, Seidman CE, Smith JD, Breslow JL, Brinton EA. Alcohol consumption raises HDL cholesterol levels by increasing the transport rate of apolipoproteins A-I and A-II. Circulation 2000; 102:2347-2352.

Cheuvront SN. The zone diet phenomenon: a closer look at the science behind the claims. Journal of the American College of Nutrition 2003; 22(1): 9-17.

Stegeman C, Kunselman B, CmClure E, Pacak D. fad diets: Implications for oral health care treatment. Access 2006; 30-35.

Yusuf S, Hawken S, Ôunpuu S, Bautista L, Grazia Franzosi M, Commerford P, Lang CC, Rumboldt Z, Onen CL, Lishen L, Tanamsup S, Wangai P, Razak F, Sharma AM, Anand SS, and on behalf of the INTERHEART Study Investigators. Obesity and the risk of myocardial infarction in 27000 participants from 52 countries: a case-control study. Lancet 2005; 366:1640-1649.

Berrington de Gonzalez A, Hartge P, Cerhan JR, Flint AJ, Hannam L, MacInnis RJ, Moore SC, Tobias GS, Anton-Culver H, Freeman LB, Beeson WL, clip SL, English DR, Folsom AR, Freedman DM, Giles G, Hakansson N, Henderson KD, Hoffman-Bolton J, Hoppin JA, Koenig KL, Lee IM, Linet MS, Park Y, Pocobelli G, Schatzkin A, Sesso HD, Weiderpass E, Wilcox BJ, Wolk A, Zeleniuch-Jacquotte A, Willett WC, Thun MJ. Body-Mass index and mortality among 1.46 million white adults. N Engl J Med 2010; 363:2211-9.

Marshall DA, Walizer EM, Vernalis MN. Achievement of heart health characteristics through participation in an intensive lifestyle change program (coronary artery disease reversal study). J Cardio Rehab Prev 2009; 29:84-94.

Niemann B, Chem Y, Teschner M, Li L, Silber RE, Rohrbach S. Obesity induces signs of premature cardiac aging in younger paitents. *J Am Coll Card* 2011; 57(5):277-589.

Owan T, Avelar E, Morley K, Jiji R, Hall N, Krezowski J, Gallager J, Williams Z, Preece K, Gundersen N, Strong MB, Pendelton RC, Sgerson N, Cloward TV, Walker JM, Farney RJ, Gress RE, Adams TD, Hunt SC, Litwin SE. Favorable changes in cardiac geometry and function following gastric bypass surgery. *J Am Coll Card* 2011 ; 57(6):732-739.

Gallagher D, Visser M, DeMeersman RE, Spuúlveda, Baumgartner RN, Pierson RN, Harris T, Heymsfield SB. Appendicular skeletal muscle mass: effects of age, gender, and ethnicity. *J Appl Physiol* 1997; 83:229-239.

Longitudinal changes in body composition in older men and women: role of body weight change and physical activity. *An J Clin Nurt 2002; 76:473-481.*

Coggan AR, Abduljalil AM, Swanson SC, Earle MS, Farris JW, Mendenhall LA, Robitaille PM. Muscle metabolism during exercise in young and older untrained and endurance-trained men. *J Appl Physiol* 1993; 75(5):2125-2133.

Prior SJ, Roth SM, Wang X, Kammerer C, Miljkovic-gacic I, Bunker CH, Wheeler VW, Patrick AL, Zmuda JM. Genetic and environmental influences on skeletal muscle phenotypes as a function of age and sex in large, multigenerational families of African heritage. *J Appl Physiol* 2007; 103:1121-1127.

Villareal DT, Chode S, Parimi N, Sinacore DR, Hilton T, Armamento-Villareal R, Napoli N, Qualls C, Shah K. Weight loss, exercise, or both and physical function in obese older adults. *N Engl J Med* 2011; 364:1218-1229.

Moe B, Angelier F, Beeech C, Chastel O. *The Journal of Experimental Biology* 2007; 210:3407-3414.

Després, JP. Health consequences of visceral obesity. *Ann Med* 2001; 33:534-541.

Hauner H, Stangl K, Schmatz Ch, burger k, Blömer, Pfeiffer EF. Body fat distribution in men with angiographically confirmed coronary artery disease. *Atherosclerosis* 1990; 85: 203-210.

Klein S, Burke LE, Bray GA, Slair S, Allison DB, Pi-Sunyer X, Hong Y, Eckel RH. Clinical implications of obesity with specific focus on cardiovascular disease: A statement for professionals from the American heart association council on nutrition, physical activity, and metabolism: endorsed by the American college of cardiology foundation. *Circulation* 2004; 110: 2952-2967.

Nakamura T, Tokunaga K, Shimomura I, Nishida M, Yoshida S, Kotani K, Islam W, Keno Y, Kobatake T, Nagai Y, Fujioka S, Tarui S, Matsuzawa Y. Contribution of visceral fat accumulation to the development of cornonary artery disease in mon-obese men. *Atherosclerosis* 2994; 107:239-246.

Onat A, Uyarel H, Hergenc G, Karabulut A, Albayrak S, Can G. Determinants and definition of abdominal obesity as related to risk of diabetes, metabolic syndrome and coronary disease in Turkish men: A prospective cohort study. *Atherosclerosis* 2007; 191:182-190.

Vajo Z, Terry JG, Brinton EA. Increased intra-abdominal fat may lower HDL levels by increasing the fractional catabolic rate of LP A-I in postmenopausal women. *Atherosclerosis* 2002; 160:495-501.

Lakka TA, Lakka HM, Salonen R, Kaplan GA, Salonen JT. Abdominal obesity is associated with accelerated progression of carotid atherosclerosis in men. *Atherosclerosis* 2001; 154:496-504.

Barlow SE and the Expert Committee. Expert committee recommendations regarding the prevention, assessment, and treatment of child and adolescent overweight and obesity: summary report. Pediatrics 2007;120 Supplement December 2007:S164—S192.

Freedman DS, Mei Z, Srinivasan SR, Berenson GS, Dietz WH. Cardiovascular risk factors and excess adiposity among overweight children and adolescents: the Bogalusa Heart Study. J Pediatr. 2007; 150(1):12—17.e2.

Whitlock EP, Williams SB, Gold R, Smith PR, Shipman SA. Screening and interventions for childhood overweight: a summary of evidence for the US Preventive Services Task Force. Pediatrics. 2005; 116(1):e125—144.

Han JC, Lawlor DA, Kimm SY. Childhood obesity. Lancet. May 15 2010; 375 (9727):1737—1748.

Dietz W. Health consequences of obesity in youth: Childhood predictors of adult disease. Pediatrics 1998; 101:518—525.

Swartz MB and Puhl R. Childhood obesity: a societal problem to solve. Obesity Reviews 2003; 4(1):57—71.

Biro FM, Wien M. Childhood obesity and adult morbidities. Am J Clin Nutr. May 2010; 91(5):1499S—1505S.

Whitaker RC, Wright JA, Pepe MS, Seidel KD, Dietz WH. Predicting obesity in young adulthood from childhood and parental obesity. N Engl J Med 1997; 37(13):869—873.

Serdula MK, Ivery D, Coates RJ, Freedman DS. Williamson DF. Byers T. Do obese children become obese adults? A review of the literature. Prev Med 1993; 22:167—177.

National Institutes of Health. Clinical Guidelines on the Identification, Evaluation, and Treatment of Overweight and Obesity in Adults: the Evidence Report. Bethesda, MD: National Institutes of Health, U.S. Department of Health and Human Services; 1998.

Freedman DS, Khan LK, Dietz WH, Srinivasan SR, Berenson GS. Relationship of childhood overweight to coronary heart disease risk factors in adulthood: The Bogalusa Heart Study. Pediatrics 2001; 108:712—718.

Nissen SE, Nicholls SJ, Wolski Kathey; et al. Effect of Rimonabant on progression of atherosclerosis in patients with abdominal obesity and coronary artery disease: The STRADIVARIUS randomized controlled trial. *JAMA* 2008; 299(13):1547-1560.

Gianni P, Jan KJ, Douglas MJ, Stuart PM, Tarnopolsky MA. Oxidative stress and the mitochondrial theory of aging in human skeletal muscle. *Experimental Gerontology* 2001; 39:1391-1400.

Little JP, Phillips SM. Resistance exercise and nutrition to counteract muscle wasting. *Appl Physiol Nut Metab* 2009; 34: 817-828.

Fujimoto T, Kemppainen J, Kalliokoski KK, Nuutila P, Ito M, Knuuti Juhani. Skeletal muscle glucose uptake response to exercise in trained and untrained men. *J Am Coll Sports Medicine* 2003:777-783.

Batty GD, Li Q, Czernichow S, Neal B, Zoungas S, Huxley R, Patel An, de Galan Bastiaan E, Woodward m, Hamet P, Harrap

SB, Poulter N, Chalmers J. Erectile dysfunction and later cardiovascular disease in men with type 2 diabetes. Russo C, Jin Zhezhen, Homma S, Rundek T, elking MS, Sacco RL, Di Tullio MR. Effect of obesity and overweight on left ventricular diastolic function. *J AM Coll Card* 2011; 57(12)1368-1374.

Sharp TA, Bell ML, Grunwald GK, Schmitz KH, Sidney S, Lewis CE, Tolan K, Hill JO. Differences in resting metabolic rate between white and African-American young adults. *Obesity research* 2002; 10(8):727-732.

Johnstone AM, Murison SD, Duncan JA, Rance KA, Speakman JR. Factors influencing variation in basal metabolic rate include fat-free mass, fat mass, age, and circulating thyroxine but not sex, circulation leptin, or triiodothyronine. *Am J Clin Nutr* 2005; 82:941-948.

Hsia J, MacFadyen JG, Monyak J, Ridker PM. Cardiovascular event reduction and adverse events among subjects attaining low-density lipoprotein cholesterol <50 mg/dl with rosuvastatin. *J AM Coll Card* 2011; 57(16)1666-1675.

Josic J, Tholen Olsson A, Wickenberg J, Lindstedt S, Hlebowicz J. "Does green tea affect postprandial glucose, insulin and satiety in healthy subjects: a randomized controlled trial." *Nutrition Journal* 9:63, 30 November 2010.

Trueb RM. Pharmacologic interventions in aging hair. *Clin Interv Aging* 2006; 1(2):121-129.

Risk of erectile dysfunction induced by arsenic exposure through well water consumption in Taiwan. Hsieh FI, Hwang TS, Hsieh YC, Lo HC, Su CT, Hsu HS, Chiou HY, Chen CJ. School of Public Health, Topnotch Stroke Research Center, Taipei Medical University, Taipei 110, Taiwan

Montague DK, Jarow JP, Broderick GA et al., "Chapter 1: The management of erectile dysfunction: an AUA update". 2005; *J. Urol.* 174 (1): 230–9.

Schrader S, Breitenstein M, Clark J, Lowe B, Turner T, Nocturnal penile tumescence and rigidity testing in bicycling patrol officers. 2002; *J Androl* 23 (6): 927–34.

Sexual Function in Men Older than 50 Years of Age, annals.org, August 5, 2003

Bujdos, Brian. New Topical Erectile Dysfunction Drug Vitaros Approved in Canada; Approved Topical Drug Testim Proves Helpful for Erectile Dysfunction. http://www.accessrx.com/blog/current-health-news/vitaros-testim-topical-drugs-treat-erectile-dysfunction-a1115. Retrieved 15 April 2011.

American vein and aesthetic institute, "Intra-Corporeal Injections for Erectile Dysfunction." http://www.medrehab.com/ICI_Impotence.php

Montague DK, Jarow JP, Broderick GA et al... "Chapter 1: The management of erectile dysfunction: an AUA update." July, 2005. *J. Urol.* 174 (1): 230–9.

Choi, Dong Mi; Park, Sangaeh; Yoon, Tae Hyung; Jeong, Hye Kyoung; Pyo, Jae Sung; Park, Janghyun; Kim, Deukjoon; Kwon, Sung Won. Determination of analogs of sildenafil and vardenafil in foods by column liquid chromatography with a photodiode array detector, mass spectrometry, and nuclear magnetic resonance spectrometry. 2008; *Journal of AOAC International* 91 (3): 580–588.

Hidden Risks of Erectile Dysfunction "Treatments" Sold Online, United States Food and Drug Administration, February 21, 2009.

Kendirci M, Nowfar S, Hellstrom WJ. "The impact of vascular risk factors on erectile function." 2005; Drugs Today (Barc) 41 (1): 65–74.

Clayton AH, Ninan PT. Depression or menopause? Presentation and management of major depressive disorder in perimenopausal and postmenopausal women. *Primary Care Companion J Clin*

Psychiatry 2010; 21(1).Slevec J, Tiggemann M. Attitudes toward cosmetic surgery in middle-aged women: Body image, aging anxiety, and the media. *Psychol Women Quart* 2010; 34:65-74.

Kouvonen, A, Stafford M, De Vogli R, Shipley MJ, Marmot MG, Cox T, Vahtera J, Väänänen A, Heponiemi T, Singh-Manoux A, Kivimäki M. Negative aspects of close relationships as a predictor of increased body mass index and waist circumference: The Whitehall II Study. *Am J Public Health* 2011; 101:1474-80.

Kegel exercise: A how-to guide for women. Mayo Clinic [Internet]. [Updated 2010 Jul 10; Retrieved 2011 Dec 27]. Available from: http://www.mayoclinic.com/health/kegel-exercises/WO00119

Aging skin care tips. Healthy-aging-for-women-babyboomers.com [Internet]. [Retrieved 2011 Dec 27]. Available from: http://www.healthy-aging-for-women-babyboomers.com/aging-skin.html

Sexuality in later life. AgePage [Internet]. National Institute on Aging. [Updated 2009 Jul; Retrieved 2011 Dec 27]. Available from: http://www.nia.nih.gov/sites/default/files/84106NIAAgePageSexin LaterLifeSINGLES09AUG212_0.pdf

Grufferman, BH. Life after 50: Women's worst fear after 50? It's not what you think. *Huffington Post* [Internet]. [Updated 2011 May 15; Retrieved 2011 Dec 27]. Available from: http://www.huffingtonpost.com/barbara-hannah-grufferman/life-after-50-womens-wors_b_861659.html

Cohen DA, Babey SH.Candy the cash register-A risk factor for obesity and chronic disease.20012 *N Engl J Med* 367;15:1381-1383.

Pomeranz JL, Brownell KD. Portion sizes and beyond-Government's legal authority to regulate food-industry practices. 20012 *N Engl J Med* 367;15:1383-1385.

Qi Q, Chu AY, Kang JH, Jensen KM, Curhan GC, Pasquale LR, Ridker PM, Hunter DJ, Willett WC, Rimm EB, Chasman DL, Hu FB, Qi L. Sugar-sweetened beverages and genetic risk of obesity. 20012 *N Engl J Med* 367; 15:1387-1396.

De Ruyter JC, Olthof MR, Seidell JC, Katan MB. A trial of sugar-free or sugar-sweetened beverates and body weight in children. 2012 *N Engl J Med* 367; 15:13971406.